I'M STILL HERE

I'M STILL HERE

a breakthrough approach

to understanding someone

living with alzheimer's

John Zeisel, Ph.D.

Avery
a member of Penguin Group (USA) Inc.
New York

Published by the Penguin Group
Penguin Group (USA) Inc., 375 Hudson Street, New York, New York 10014, USA ·
Penguin Group (Canada), 90 Eglinton Avenue East, Suite 700, Toronto, Ontario
M4P 2Y3, Canada (a division of Pearson Canada Inc.) · Penguin Books Ltd,
80 Strand, London WC2R 0RL, England · Penguin Ireland, 25 St Stephen's Green, Dublin 2,
Ireland (a division of Penguin Books Ltd) · Penguin Group (Australia),
250 Camberwell Road, Camberwell, Victoria 3124, Australia
(a division of Pearson Australia Group Pty Ltd) · Penguin Books India Pvt Ltd,
11 Community Centre, Panchsheel Park, New Delhi–110 017, India ·
Penguin Group (NZ), 67 Apollo Drive, Rosedale, North Shore 0632, New Zealand
(a division of Pearson New Zealand Ltd) · Penguin Books (South Africa) (Pty) Ltd,
24 Sturdee Avenue, Rosebank, Johannesburg 2196, South Africa

Penguin Books Ltd, Registered Offices: 80 Strand, London WC2R 0RL, England

Most Avery books are available at special quantity discounts for bulk purchase for sales promotions, premiums, fund-
raising, and educational needs. Special books or book excerpts also can be created to fit specific needs. For
details, write Penguin Group (USA) Inc. Special Markets, 375 Hudson Street, New York, NY 10014.

Library of Congress Cataloging-in-Publication Data
Zeisel, John.
I'm still here : a breakthrough approach to understanding someone living with Alzheimer's / John Zeisel.
p.   cm.
Includes bibliographical references and index.
ISBN 978-1-58333-335-8
1. Alzheimer's disease—Patients—Care.   I. Title.
RC523.Z45   2009   2008046233
616.8'31—dc22

Printed in the United States of America
1   3   5   7   9   10   8   6   4   2

BOOK DESIGN BY TANYA MAIBORODA

Neither the publisher nor the author is engaged in rendering professional advice or services to the individual
reader. The ideas, procedures, and suggestions in this book are not intended as a substitute for consulting with a
physician. All matters regarding health require medical supervision. Neither the author nor the publisher shall be
liable or responsible for any loss or damage allegedly arising from any information or suggestion in this book.

Outdoor recreational activities are by their very nature potentially hazardous. All participants in such activities
must assume the responsibility for their own actions and safety. If you have any health problems or medical conditions, consult with your physician before undertaking any outdoor activities. The information in this book cannot replace sound judgment and good decision making, which can help reduce risk exposure, nor does the scope
of this book allow for disclosure of all the potential hazards and risks involved in such activities. Learn as much as
possible about the outdoor recreational activities in which you participate, prepare for the unexpected, and be
cautious. The reward will be a safer and more enjoyable experience.

While the author has made every effort to provide accurate telephone numbers and Internet addresses at the time
of publication, neither the publisher nor the author assumes any responsibility for errors, or for changes that occur
after publication. Further, the publisher does not have any control over and does not assume any responsibility for
author or third-party websites or their content.

For all the residents, families, staff, and colleagues
at Hearthstone Alzheimer Care and the
Hearthstone Alzheimer's Foundation
who have helped turn an idea
and a dream into a reality,
and from whom I have
learned so much.

CONTENTS

AUTHOR'S NOTE

☙ IF YOU would like to share your story with me and others, please e-mail it to MyStory@ImStillHere.org. You are invited to share experiences through which you have been touched by compassion; responses to following the mindfulness meditation I describe at the end of the book; and insights you have reached as a partner—what I call the gifts of Alzheimer's.

My blog is available at www.ImStillHere.org, as are reproductions of paintings and other visual material referred to in this book.

1

EMBRACING ALZHEIMER'S

a new philosophy
of care

Why is it that some ideas or behaviors or products start epidemics and others don't? And what can we do to deliberately start and control positive epidemics of our own?
—MALCOLM GLADWELL

I FIRST became interested in the challenges of helping people living with Alzheimer's when about fifteen years ago a nursing home operator approached me for program and design advice. My background is in environmental design, and he came to me because so many of the Alzheimer's beds in his special-care unit were empty. At that time I didn't realize this would become my life's work. It did, because the rather dry question introduced me to a field waiting for redefinition.

My grandfather, whom we called "Apus," lived with us on the Upper West Side of Manhattan. We called him "senile" and took it for granted that he was a member of the family with certain abilities, and there were some things we didn't ask of him. I never thought of his condition as an illness. That was the old way.

Today, in North America alone there are 5 million people living with Alzheimer's, each with an average of five care partners— making 25 million care partners. Worldwide, these figures leap to 50 million people living with Alzheimer's and 250 million care partners. The care of such people has become a major medical industry, with the number of nursing homes rapidly expanding, and with Alzheimer's drugs sold in the billions annually. Existing drugs and those in the pipeline that provide hope to future generations at best delay the disease a few months or years; they do not eliminate it. The prognosis for the future: many more people living even longer in the early stages of Alzheimer's than today.

I have learned over the last fifteen years that treating people with Alzheimer's the old way was often better, whether they live at home, in assisted-living residences, or in nursing homes. In order to treat people living with Alzheimer's as people rather than as patients, we first have to appreciate their capabilities as well as their losses. We need to see the person through the fog of the illness, and we have to employ as many nonpharmacological treatments as pharmaceutical ones.

I have stayed in this field because I gradually realized how much the lessons I have learned about people living with Alzheimer's apply to others with physical, sensory, and cognitive disabilities. The treatment principles involved are equally valid for autism, mental illness, mental retardation, manic depression, diabetes, HIV, and even for a simple cold, or a twisted knee. In fact, the fundamental treatment principles that I describe in this book are universal.

The people living with Alzheimer's have also inspired me to stay in the field. The way the illness affects the brain leaves most of them exceptionally perceptive, increasingly creative, and highly emotionally intelligent for years.

I have developed and tested these theories over the last decade and a half, running Alzheimer's assisted-living treatment residences in Massachusetts and New York. We call them "treatment" centers because the physical environment, the communication, and the programs all independently act to reduce residents' symptoms, including agitation, anxiety, aggression, and apathy. *I'm Still Here* is the result of the lessons learned from this group of people and the commitment I have made to spread this optimistic message.

This book strongly acknowledges that no one welcomes living with Alzheimer's, and that to date there is no cure. Nevertheless, *I'm Still Here* looks at the positive side of this illness: the half-full rather than the half-empty glass. I advocate treating people living with Alzheimer's as "people" first and then as those with an illness. I advocate including people living with Alzheimer's in society—at museums and theaters, among other places. I explain that people usually live with Alzheimer's for over a decade and that for much of that time they can function with less help than most people think, can enjoy themselves, and can even learn new things. As important, the people who care for them can maintain positive relationships and share vibrant memories for the entire course of the illness through photos, music, art, personal stories, and visits to museums and other community cultural events.

I'm Still Here is an invitation to a different worldview based on the realities of the big picture—the fact that there is no cure in the near future; the fact that millions of people living with Alzheimer's can live active lives rather than being institutionalized and hidden from society; the fact that how partners see the illness—positively or negatively—has a major impact on the partner with the illness.

This book carries two frequently overlooked uncommon commonsense messages.

1. The skills and capacities of people living with Alzheimer's that don't diminish over time, or do so more slowly, provide windows for connection and communication.
2. Through those windows lie opportunities to establish and build new and vibrant relationships that can sustain us and them over time, supporting both care and well-being.

Embracing and translating these two messages requires that we understand the following:

- Love is a universal language understood far into the illness, even to the end of life. If everyone involved with the illness learns to say "I love you" to the other, the other person will understand and be more present and relationships can grow.

- Everyone has preexisting, instinctual abilities that building a caring relationship can capitalize on, such as our ability to understand music, facial expressions, and human touch—the meaning of a song, a smile, and a hug. Drawing on these innate abilities enables everyone living with Alzheimer's to function better than expected, because they are never lost.

- Memories are not held in just one part of the brain into which we place them like a DVD disk for later retrieval. Rather, we place attributes of experience in various parts of the brain—faces in one part, colors in another, emotions related to the experience in another. Later, a brain function that acts like a call to Scotty in *Star Trek*—"Beam me up, Scotty"—retrieves them. Art, music, environment, and Alzheimer's-competent communication help those memories reappear, just as Scotty helps Captain Kirk and his crew reassemble aboard the *Enterprise.*

- Alzheimer's is treatable, and the best treatment is one that carefully balances nonpharmacological with pharmacological approaches. Nonpharmacological treatment includes carefully planning and managing both the social and physical environment of the person.

- It is important that all caregivers burdened with guilt remind themselves that Alzheimer's is an organic illness of the brain, and that sharing care-partnering tasks with others is keeping a promise, not breaking it.

- Partners get sick more often than do the people they care for: Those who care for people living with Alzheimer's tend not to take care of themselves. They tend to get sick more often and for longer periods than the people they care for. Taking care of oneself is the surest way to help the person you love.

- People living with Alzheimer's live in the present moment. Mindfulness of being in the present moment ourselves is a first step toward being in the mind of a person living with Alzheimer's. Being totally present to our own breath through meditation can help us experience that fleeting moment— the Alzheimer's experience. This is as close as we can possibly get to being where we are and to being in the same place as the person we love who is living with Alzheimer's.

Many people as they grow older forget one thing or another. This is not Alzheimer's. *I'm Still Here* provides a human understanding of the profound changes the person with Alzheimer's is going through. This understanding alone is the greatest defense against the fear we all live with—a fear that the research and other fund-raising communities unfortunately promote in their desire for funding. Understanding also leads to compassion—a necessary ingredient for treating oneself well and for being able to give of oneself to the other person throughout the illness.

A life with Alzheimer's can be seen as a glass mostly full or completely empty—and each is a state of mind. This book lays out a positive view of living with Alzheimer's that can lead to a life with quality for all involved as well as to effective treatment. The Alzheimer's glass is more than half full in this book.

A person living with Alzheimer's is first "a person" and only then someone with a disease. The way the world sees Alzheimer's today is that a person is almost totally lost once he or she receives an Alzheimer's diagnosis—lost both to themselves and to those who love them. An Alzheimer's diagnosis is seen as an Alzheimer's "sentence." But this just isn't so. Throughout the more than decade-long progress of the disease, the person is crying out, "I'm still here." We all need to start hearing that cry before it fades away completely.

This book describes how much remains alive and vital in the brain of a person living with Alzheimer's disease and shows how certain parts of the brain even enable someone living with the disease to function more sensitively than before.

If we rely primarily on drugs to alleviate the symptoms of Alzheimer's—or what most people assume to be those symptoms—there is little available treatment at present. Some cognitive enhancement drugs have some effects; many have side effects. Some mood drugs can reduce disturbing behaviors, often at the price of reduced quality of life.

In order to assess the impacts of medications and of non-pharmacological treatments on Alzheimer's symptoms, we need first to agree on what are symptoms and what are not. For example, we know that one symptom of Alzheimer's is difficulty dealing with complex situations, and that when a person faces these difficulties, she often gets frustrated, agitated, and sometimes aggressive. The symptom is loss of executive function in the brain's frontal lobes and the concomitant difficulty dealing with complex events. The other effects are actually secondary or tertiary symptoms, if they can even be called symptoms at all. In the next chapter I articulate these differences and explain how important it is to see them, in order to be able to develop treatments that work and for partners to develop meaningful relationships with the people living with Alzheimer's.

Nonpharmacological environmental and behavioral treatments can have dramatic results with few side effects. Symptoms that everyone thought were integral to the disease can be reduced. There is a new message to be heard: "People living with Alzheimer's are still people. Alzheimer's is treatable. Don't give up."

At this point, readers might understandably ask, "What do you mean, 'Don't give up'!?" So much of what we hear and read and see about Alzheimer's paints those living with the illness as unable to cope with their environment, unable to relate to others, and having lost their sense of self. But to build healthy relationships with those living with Alzheimer's, each of us has to connect through those capacities and facilities that don't diminish with the progression of the disease, or at least diminish most gradually. When we listen to music or visit a museum together, we are building such relationships. We are also reducing the secondary and tertiary symptoms of Alzheimer's. Those living with Alzheimer's who use parts of their brains that still function well, feel enabled and competent, and are less apathetic, agitated, anxious, and aggressive.

Alzheimer's is presented in a totally negative light not only in modern advertisements and films, but also in classic literature. Although Shakespeare didn't know at the time that he was writing about Alzheimer's, he held the same view. At the end of Jaques's well-known seven-ages-of man speech in act 2 of *As You Like It*, Shakespeare refers obliquely to living with Alzheimer's disease in old age as a return to the state of "childishness and mere oblivion":

> *All the world's a stage,*
> *And all the men and women merely players:*
> *They have their exits and their entrances;*
> *And one man in his time plays many parts,*
> *His acts being seven ages. At first the infant,*
> *Mewling and puking in the nurse's arms. . . .*

Last scene of all,
That ends this strange eventful history,
Is second childishness and mere oblivion,
Sans teeth, sans eyes, sans taste, sans everything.

While this is beautifully poetic, it is not accurate. It is easy to count the ways that the analogy between Alzheimer's and child-hood is inaccurate. A child has limited history and memories, while people in old age with or without Alzheimer's have a long history of experience. They have lived through several historical eras, in various cities and perhaps countries, and they have ex-perienced the world changing around them in major ways. They have seen technology develop, and political upheaval. Most have children and grandchildren. They know how to repair bro-ken objects, cook, build houses, teach, write, paint, play piano, knit—to name a few of the things that they can do that children can't. They have profound personal life experiences. Some have fought in wars, marched for peace, suffered in concentration camps, or moved from the countries of their birth as refugees. They have held responsible jobs and achieved accolades for their achievements. They definitely are not like children.

Another inaccurate perception is that when people are diag-nosed with Alzheimer's they have no future—that an Alzheimer's diagnosis is an Alzheimer's sentence. The condition lasts ten to fifteen years, a time span that definitely constitutes a future. "What kind of future is it if people can't remember their children and where they are?" those who don't understand the disease ask. That question assumes that memories are gone, which they are not, they are just increasingly inaccessible without some help. It also assumes that the future is based in the past and in past memories. It is not. The future is based on many present moments—moments the person experiences fully every day and every minute. The future for people living with Alzheimer's promotes new relationships, quality of life, and joy. To see the future in this way requires us to realize that the person living with Alzheimer's is a new person with reference to the old person he always was—but that he is not that person any longer. Neither can our relationships be the same. While the person still cares for us and continues to love us and we them, we must have new expectations and build a new relationship. The first step is to discard old expectations and role relationships that limit our ability to see the person and relate to him or her in a new way.

The person herself as well as every family member holds a key to keeping the whole family's story going into the future. Each family member holds one key to the person's past, present, and future. Each person knows and can share with others the major themes and scenes in her life that are likely to be embedded in memory. When family members are present, she knows who each person is and she remembers herself—even if she may not be able every time to remember a name or a specific relationship. Family members know how to read the moods and body language of the person they love; they know how to provide joy and quality of life better than anyone; and they are the key to identifying the ongoing narrative. And in return, the person living with Alzheimer's knows her family members' moods and body language. This is a mutual process of understanding that does not end with a diagnosis.

Every family member and close partner of someone living with Alzheimer's has experienced the person asking, "Who are you?" or repeating a question he asked and that was answered just a few minutes before. "He's lost his memory," people say to themselves. Yes, he has a problem remembering certain things that his brain prevents him from embedding into long-term memory. Chapter 3 describes the brain regions that one must understand to reach the person behind Alzheimer's—those regions that are affected most, and those that hold promise for building strong relationships because they are less affected.

Recalling a name or a recently posed question is really a small part of his or any of our memories. What about emotional memories of happy and sad times that can't be expressed in words? What about the lasting smile when his granddaughter hugs him and tells him how much she loves him? Among the memories lodged in his brain are the following types, each of which provides the opportunity for communication and understanding.

MEMORIES STILL THERE

SENSE MEMORIES

Smell/fragrance memory

Touch memory

Visual memory

Body memory

Music memory

Taste memory

Sound memory

Proprioceptive body memory

EMOTIONAL MEMORIES

Times of joy

Sad memories

Fear memory

Pain memory

Love memories

Excitement

Regret

Shock

Compassion

BODY MEMORIES

Having a baby

Riding a bicycle

Throwing a baseball

Putting a golf ball

Dancing the fox-trot

Breaking a leg

Carrying a heavy load

SKILL MEMORIES

Cooking

Dancing

Drawing

Knitting

Bowling

Sewing

Digging

HARDWIRED MEMORIES

The sun

Smiles

Fireplace

ART MEMORY

Paintings

Poetry

Music

Sculpture

Dance

ENVIRONMENTAL MEMORY	**AUTOBIOGRAPHICAL MEMORIES**
Color	Life period memories (child-
Place	hood, school, teenage years)
Object	Type of events—hunting, going
Texture	to the beach, chopping
Environmental mood memory	firewood
Spatial memory	Special event memories
	Family memories—my wedding,
	my son's college graduation
SONG MEMORIES	**STORY MEMORIES**
Popular tunes	How I met my wife/husband
Religious hymns	When I was a child—that time
Children's songs	of life
Military music	Childhood events
Dance Music	When I saw my first movie
	Fairy tales
COLLECTIVE MEMORIES— MAJOR EVENTS EXPERIENCED	**SOCIAL NORMS MEMORY**
World War II	How to be polite to others at
D-day	dinner
The great NYC blackout	How to greet someone coming
Elvis Presley on	to visit
The Ed Sullivan Show	How to behave at holiday
The assassination of	parties
President Kennedy	How to behave at religious
9/11	ceremonies
	How to behave at a wedding
	Just how to say hello

TIP-OF-THE-TONGUE MEMORY Names you know but you can't recall *without a cue*	**HABIT MEMORY (LEARNING)** Eating with chopsticks Putting eyeglasses in the same spot every night Setting a table the same way every time

THE FOLLOWING MEMORY TYPES ARE MORE COMPROMISED THAN THOSE ABOVE.

COGNITIVE MAP/WAY-FINDING MEMORY "I know where I am when I'm there, I know where I am going if I can see my destination, and I know where I was going when I get there." Getting to the bathroom at night without a light Finding your way back to a childhood haunt Getting home from wherever you are	**FACTUAL (LEARNED) MEMORY** Things I "know" (e.g., the names of presidents, grandchildren's birthdays) Test memory—cram-for-an-exam memory
COMPLEX SEQUENCE MEMORY Brushing one's teeth Organizing a meal Cooking a complex meal Getting dressed Putting a diaper on a baby Packing for a trip	**MESSAGE MEMORY** Remembering what was just said Remembering a person you met recently only once Remembering a phone message just left with you A phone call you just finished A phone number

All these memories except those at the end of the list are readily accessible to people living with Alzheimer's and their partners. And message memory, factual learning, way-finding, and complex sequence memory can be accessed with appropriate approaches and communication.

As people age with Alzheimer's they retain certain memories better than others. Some may be skills that are so ingrained they express themselves without the person's thinking, such as knitting, hammering together two pieces of wood, putting a golf ball, or playing a musical instrument. Others may be hardwired in our brains, such as caring for another person in a time of need, seeing meaning in a work of art, or tapping rhythmically to music. Whatever the remaining skills, everyone has them and everyone can be engaged if these skills are appealed to kindly and sensitively.

Visiting a friend's ex-mother-in-law recently, we remarked at the beautifully knitted sweater she was wearing. She told us she had knitted it and that she always knitted sweaters for her sons when they were growing up. My friend, who knits quite well, readily announced that she liked knitting but needed help to improve. From then on, visits included a short knitting lesson. My friend brought the knitting needles, a skein of wool, and her desire to know more. Her ex-mother-in-law drew on her knitting skills and her deeply rooted sense of caring for another person to teach new stitches. The remaining memories of these encounters served to cement the new relationship the two old friends developed.

Everyone has his own unique capabilities. These may include reading the newspaper out loud to others, singing, gardening, or dancing. Whatever they are, they are there and it is our job to uncover, celebrate, and embrace them so that everyone living with Alzheimer's, no matter where in the progress of the illness they are, maintains their dignity, independence, and self-respect.

People living with Alzheimer's also retain critical powers of observation even though they may have difficulty being reflective about what they see. When faced with an objective situation, the person at all stages of Alzheimer's can describe with great clarity what she sees. She is not burdened, as many others are, with reflective self-critical thoughts such as "Should I say that?" or "Is that the right thing to say in this situation?" The ability to observe and appreciate makes people living with Alzheimer's wonderful listeners and wonderful companions. They see so much that we take for granted and thus overlook, whether walking in the park or through a shopping mall. They have interesting and often funny things to say. The person you love who is living with this illness is a wonderful companion.

People living with Alzheimer's are artists, performers, and an attentive audience. An artist expresses himself from his heart, avoids being overly self-critical, and can unselfconsciously express his "self" in his art. The lack of a fully functioning brain "comparer" makes many people living with Alzheimer's better artists than they were before the disease. Just as inventive artistic personalities who have little regard for rules of society are not deterred from their creative goals even in the face of obvious difficulties, people living with Alzheimer's are often freer, more honest, and more expressive than most others.

The Artists for Alzheimer's program (ARTZ) described in chapter 4 is a multifaceted program that enables people living with Alzheimer's and their partners to take advantage of such special creative abilities. One fascinating dimension of the artistic abilities that people living with Alzheimer's reveals—derived in large part from their canny ability to be present to where they are, to just "be there"—is that those abilities express themselves in both art appreciation and art creation. The insights people living with Alzheimer's bring to the paintings they see at museums are as interesting, amusing, and artistic as are the drawings and paintings they create as part of ARTZ. When they are faced with an artistic experience, these perceptive skills emerge eloquently.

Observing Toulouse-Lautrec's *La Goulue at the Moulin Rouge* ("The Glutton") on a special tour for people with Alzheimer's that my colleague Sean Caulfield and I developed at the Museum of Modern Art, several participants instinctively commented on the roughness of the "man" on the left pulling the woman out of the bar, although the person on the left is wearing a dress and has long hair or a wig. Close observation reveals the person's thick hands and masculine features. Oscar Wilde, the famous play-wright, was visiting Lautrec at the time he painted *La Goulue,* and this character—ostensibly La Goulue's sister—might well be an homage to Wilde. Art history books chronicle viewers' outrage at Lautrec including such a rough-looking person in this painting. Participants' discussion about the roughness and gender of the fig-ure, paralleling art critics' comments, is one of many insightful ob-servations people living with Alzheimer's make in such situations.

As an audience for the work of other artists—paintings, po-etry, theater, music, circus acts, short films—people living with Alzheimer's are equally present and nonjudgmental. They are all artists. As Marily Cintra, an Australian artist and culture consul-tant, said to me after we discussed this subject: "Now I under-stand why I am so relaxed around people living with Alzheimer's. They are as artistic as I am."

In chapters 4 and 5, I describe how visual and dramatic arts—museum exhibitions, music, theater, film, and the circus arts—touch people living with Alzheimer's in ways no other experience does. Art experiences enable them to focus for longer periods, to perceive and express their perceptions, and to access both long- and short-term memories. Art of all sorts also enables people living with Alzheimer's and those without it to focus together on something outside themselves, rather than on each other. Such shared experi-ences bring everyone closer together and serve as a basis for build-ing new and strong relationships, the topic of chapters 7 and 8.

While art experiences draw out people's skills and abilities and bring partners together, so do the physical environments in which they live. Design for people living with Alzheimer's, the topic of chapter 6, supports their independence. It helps them know the limits of where they are safe, know where they are going, know what is their own place and what to do when they are together with others. Design for people living with Alzheimer's reduces the secondary symptoms of the illness—those that are not directly caused by changes to the brain, including apathy, anxiety, agitation, and aggression that to a large degree are not caused by the disease. Rather, they are caused by a person living in a place that is frustrating and difficult to negotiate. In chapter 6, I discuss the design principles that support the well-being of those living with Alzheimer's:

- Camouflaging and otherwise reducing the importance of exits leading to dangerous places.
- Providing destinations at the end of pathways so people walk rather than wander.
- Providing people with a place of their own with their own possessions that reinforce their sense of themselves.
- Common spaces decorated and sized to communicate what the appropriate behaviors are for those areas.
- Gardens designed therapeutically, and with safety in mind, so that residents know what time it is and what season it is.

- Making the place like a home so that people living there with Alzheimer's feel at home.
- Making certain that all the sensory inputs—colors, sounds, textures—are those that residents understand easily.
- Supportive environments that enable everyone there to do what they can by themselves.

Art, environmental design, and music reflect the message of personhood that is clearly there to be heard. People living with Alzheimer's let you know what they think—clearly and often. They might not use the same words to express themselves as highly left-brain people might, but they can be just as eloquent. Later in the Alzheimer's journey, the expressions may be in their smiles or furrowed brows, in their body language, in the way they embrace you, or in the glint of recognition in their eyes when they see certain people again. It is too easy to classify those who have lived with Alzheimer's for many years as nonpeople because they might no longer relate to the world the same way they used to, or as we think we do. Discarding people in this way reduces their quality of life and ours. We burden them with disregard and loneliness. We burden ourselves with "having to visit" again and again with nothing to say and do—just wait until it's time to leave and resume our lives.

The dozen or more years living with Alzheimer's are marked by different levels of cognitive ability and impairment. During that time, and especially in the early stages, everyone living with this disease is capable of meaningful relationships, perceptions, feelings, and involvement in life. Why does society shunt these people away, rather than find ways to involve them in our lives and our communities? One reason for this is our own ignorance of how to build a relationship with someone going through the changes associated with Alzheimer's. Everyone who loves and takes care of a person living with Alzheimer's faces what appear to be insurmountable odds in developing a new relationship with that person as she or he changes. Despite these fears, every relationship between a person and someone that person loves who has Alzheimer's can still be vibrant and rewarding—even improved from earlier relationships—but only if both people first get to know each other again.

The new relationship each person establishes can be mutual; with both partner and person living with Alzheimer's expressing their needs and having the other respond. Everyone who learns to say "I love you" to the other can have such a relationship, because love is a universal language understood far into the illness, even to the end of life.

People who want a relationship also have to learn to say "Please help me" when they reach the end of their rope. Only those who take care of themselves can be there for another person. For someone who does not have the disease, it may seem selfish to think about oneself; but it is necessary.

When traveling and at parties, because of my unique position managing assisted-living treatment residences for people living with Alzheimer's, I often find myself in conversation with people facing Alzheimer's in a family member or friend. I don't tell them they ought to build a relationship with those they know and love. Rather, I draw on their own inner knowledge to develop with them a picture of how they might engage the person behind the illness, provide meaning, and establish a positive relationship between them and the person they care about. I tailor my stories to their unique situation as a friend, a family member, a spouse, a child, or a professional—whatever their "partner" relation is. I tailor the stories to the responses the person has to our conversation.

"My mother doesn't recognize me, what can I do?" they might ask. I ask how they address their mother when they visit her. Do they say, "Hi, Mom, remember me?" which is a test of her memory, can be upsetting, and is likely to elicit the anxious response "No, who are you?" Or do they hold their mother's hand in theirs, put their face at her level, look her directly in the eye, and say, "Hi, Mom, I'm your son Alex, we have wonderful times together, and I love you very much"? Such an introduction is more likely to elicit a smile and the response "Oh, Alex, it's so nice to see you."

Or they ask, "A friend of mine just found out she has Alzheimer's. I stopped calling because she doesn't know who I am when I call. Is there anything else I can do?" "Have you also stopped going to see her?" I ask. They generally say they have stopped visiting because "what's the use?" The "use," I tell them, is that they and their memories keep their friend attached to life. I suggest they assemble a book of photographs from trips they have taken together or from an anniversary party, go over to their friend's house, introduce themselves by name, and look through the book, recalling feelings they may have had at the time and talking about the wonderful memories.

When they tell me that the person they know is too distracted to sit still, I tell them that I too have tried to get someone to look at pictures who has been nervously walking around the room, not noticing me, and crying. It is not easy to attract someone's attention who is so agitated—but it can be done. The trick is to focus your own attention intensely on the task at hand, no matter what else is happening, and to repeatedly ask for help understanding the photographs. It is a matter of will, and the person whose will is stronger generally successfully defines the situation.

When I ask them how they feel about the person, they invariably use the term "love." Expressing love to someone living with Alzheimer's is one of the keys to making and keeping contact. Being able to truthfully and openly say "I love you" to someone puts you in touch with yourself and opens the other person to you. Love is a universal, hardwired language. People understand until the end of life that by loving them you accept them for who they are.

At the end of such conversations, I acknowledge how hard it is even to think of taking such steps, because their family member or friend has changed and so has the relationship. If they can start down this path they will be giving something important to him or her, and at the same time they will reap great personal satisfaction—the gifts of Alzheimer's. I try to leave them in a more positive state of mind than when I met them, not just with tidbits of knowledge. The road to easing the burden of Alzheimer's begins with shifting one's point of view.

"I'm still here, please help me, I love you, and don't give up" is my message for those living with Alzheimer's as well as for their partners. In this book, the term "partner" refers to each person in an Alzheimer's relationship. Both the person with the illness and the other person in the relationship are partners to each other. When used to refer to an individual who regularly spends time with someone living with Alzheimer's, the term "partner" indicates a spouse, paid caregiver, friend, medical professional, social worker, or family member.

Each of us grows and changes continually. If we choose to stay connected to others as they and we change during the passage of the disease, we learn about ourselves, about relationships, and even about the meaning of life.

These are the gifts of Alzheimer's we can reap.

2

THE ALZHEIMER'S JOURNEY

the symptoms and
progression of the disease

The key biological fact that Darwin appreciated, and that has facilitated the development of animal models of anxiety states, is that anxiety—fear itself—is a universal, instinctive response to a threat to one's body or social status and is therefore critical for survival. Anxiety signals a potential threat, which requires an adaptive response. —ERIC R. KANDEL

AT THE START of the Alzheimer's journey, the person knows what is happening to her and realizes that she cannot perform up to the same expectations—both her own and others'—as she was able to in the past at work, at home, in the family, and in public. There is no place she can go to get away from struggling with everyday activities. This does not mean that the person with this awareness can't perform well in public, only that she can't do it the way she used to and the way others still expect her to. If others begin to avoid her because she's "different," she becomes even more isolated and feels even more that she is not there. When people help her celebrate her continuing abilities and successes, she can "come out of the closet" of shame and into the full light of day. She can fully be herself. As Cathleen McBride wrote in the newsletter of the Massachusetts chapter of the Alzheimer's Association shortly after being diagnosed: "I am really only beginning to enjoy the now of life, something that completely passed me by before. So, all in all, I would describe Alzheimer's as a new stage in a wonderful life, no less challenging or interesting than all the earlier stages."

Like Cathleen McBride, Richard Taylor lives with Alzheimer's. He was sixty-three years old when he wrote the message quoted below; he found out he had Alzheimer's when he was fifty-nine. His age means that he has early-onset Alzheimer's disease—a form of the illness that strikes about 10 percent of those with Alzheimer's. Before he retired, Richard taught abnormal psychology, business communication, public speaking, and interpersonal communication at Indiana University, Wayne State University, and Rice University.

Richard regularly broadcasts e-mails to friends and colleagues about his thoughts and experience living with Alzheimer's. "From time to time I get some interesting insights into myself and my disease. I think about thinking because that is what I did for a living," he writes. He is also author of *Alzheimer's from the Inside Out,* a book written from the point of view of someone going through the illness.

On January 5, 2007, Richard sent an e-mail to his six-thousand-person mailing list. The following from that e-mail makes eloquently clear that he is more than just "still here."

A Plea from All the Me's I Will Be

I was a whole person the moment I was born. I was a whole person, yes, even in my teen years. I am a whole person now. Even near death, even in death I am a full and whole person. Although thanks to Doctor Alzheimer and his sticky footed troops tromping around between my ears I now evolve, change, morph in ways neither of us can predict or understand—I am still me!

Never will I be three-fourths of a person, half of a person, nor ⅟₇₃ of a person. There has not, nor will there ever be a moment in my life when I am not a complete Human Being. Please get this; it's important to me, to those who love me, to those who are paid to care for me. It is important to our society. I am always me. . . .

Why don't people understand and appreciate the fact I am still one of them! Honest! Just not exactly like one of them— just slightly different but basically the same. . . .

Hands up in the audience if you are trying to help me be all I can be for as long as I can be? Who wants to help enable me to be as much as I want, as much I can, as much as I should be right now, and every tomorrow until the day I die? . . .

I honestly believe some people now don't see me as a whole person. Every visible symptom is a sign I am not whole. Some people see me as still whole, but it is just a matter of time until I am not, and because of that inevitability, they now feel very sorry for me. Some people see me as still whole, yet with a few missing pieces, but not enough just quite yet to declare me defective, not me. "You are still my husband, but you sometimes act different from the man I married."

They are of course all, all wrong. I am me. Not necessarily still the me you and I knew prior to the disease process, but still Me.

The fact that he has Alzheimer's is less present in the person's consciousness as the disease progresses. The person living with Alzheimer's becomes less aware of being ill. On the other hand, he remains as aware as ever of the fact that he either fits in with others socially or he doesn't. When his wife berates him for repeating himself or for forgetting a planned event he feels as bad as he ever has. He feels even worse because he may remember only with difficulty and therefore understand even less what he has done wrong and why he is being berated. He still has access to his many memories, but has a harder time directing himself to the right part of his "memory bank."

Realizing, understanding, and acting on the fact that the person is still there at this stage requires greater involvement and attention on the part of every partner in relationship with the person. Respect and dignity can be conferred by actions such as:

- *Addressing the person directly*—never referring to him indirectly when you are in his presence.
- *Subtly helping him be in control*—neatening clothes that may be out of place, quietly reminding him how to get somewhere on his own, waiting until he expresses himself rather than speaking *for* him.
- *Providing props*—keeping photographs and other mementos at hand that cue significant memories, introducing these with a phrase like "You remember little Pie-Pie, your grandson."
- *Never testing the person's memory*—never asking, "Do you remember my name?" or showing him a picture and asking, "Do you remember who this is?"

Toward the end of the journey, even when a person may have lost the ability to speak clearly and may need a lot of help walking from one side of the room to the other, the person is still there and can still be reached. She also is acutely aware of being treated with disrespect. At this point, it requires even greater discipline and love to remember the person is still there. Touching her hand or shoulder—physically—always works to make her aware that you are there, that she is there, and that you and she still have a relationship. A family member's presence is also always appreciated—even if others say the person living with Alzheimer's doesn't know you're there. She does! Music, images, perfume, and other nonverbal forms of communication let the person with the illness know that someone who cares for her realizes she is present. To hear her say or just to sense her saying, "I'm still here and thank you for knowing this," you first have to believe and be ready to hear it yourself. You need to be aware and present enough to see and respond to the signs she is giving you—a smile, a raised hand, a hug in response to a hug. You must also reflect on the nature of "personhood." Does a person have to speak intelligibly, to remember the names of the presidents of the United States, or to be independent in caring for him or herself in order to be a person?

WHAT ARE—AND WHAT AREN'T—SYMPTOMS

The symptoms of Alzheimer's are implicit in the story I just told you of how the condition tends to progress over its course. Making them explicit, however, is harder than one might think because most people tend to clump together all the behaviors associated with living with Alzheimer's in a single term—symptoms—no matter what their cause actually might be.

Insightful clinical and analytic research has been carried out that provides greater clarity on what are the primary symptoms of Alzheimer's disease, what are its secondary symptoms, and which tertiary symptoms may not be symptoms at all, but rather natural reactions to social and physical environments.

Primary Alzheimer's behavioral symptoms are directly attributable to either cognitive or functional impairments, according to Ladislav Volicer, a physician and researcher at the Veterans Administration Hospital in Bedford, Massachusetts. Cognitive impairments include difficulty accessing memories about what to do in specific situations such as how to make casual conversation at a party. Also included are problems with executive function, the capacity we have in our frontal lobes to organize complex sequences of activities, that make initiating activities difficult, as well as speech deficits that prevent a person from expressing him or herself clearly, and sometimes from understanding others. Functional deficits make it hard for some people living with Alzheimer's to use tools and utensils and thus to continue with professional skills or hobbies in the same way as in the past, and eventually making it difficult even to carry out some basic activities of daily living.

Secondary behaviors are effects of primary deficits but are not immediate reactions to them. In a stressful situation, for example, if a person who has difficulty controlling his impulses (a primary Alzheimer's symptom) strikes out aggressively, this latter behavior is a reaction to not being able to handle what is happening to him, not a primary symptom. An important distinction in terms of how people treat them is that some secondary behaviors are not disturbing to others, while some are disturbing. Apathy—being listless and uninvolved with one's surroundings—is the main non-disturbing secondary behavioral symptom. In the extreme, an apathetic person just stares into space without interacting with his social or physical environment. Others just ignore this apathetic behavior because it doesn't disturb them. What is overlooked is that apathy tends to express the person's own discomfort and low quality of life, and that involving the person in meaningful activities can treat this particular secondary symptom.

Disturbing secondary behaviors—that are not immediate consequences of primary brain impairments yet bother partners and others—fall into two types: behaviors that are *uninvoked* by physical stimuli, environments, or personal interaction, and those that are *invoked*. Uninvoked disturbing behaviors, not attributable to a clear and immediate cause, can be grouped under the general heading "agitation." Expressing agitation, according to Alzheimer's researcher Jiska Cohen-Mansfield, is one way people with Alzheimer's communicate to others that they are excited or that they feel something unpleasant. True agitation takes the form of restlessness, repetitive movement, and verbal expression and is what remains after everything has been done to reduce internal and external stimuli that might be upsetting the person.

Agitation should not be confused with invoked aggression. By involving the person in continuous activity, you can reduce or eliminate agitated behaviors. Reducing aggression requires eliminating its cause.

Aggression is not a disease symptom, at least not for most types of Alzheimer's and dementia. It is a natural reaction on the part of the person living with Alzheimer's to feeling that another person is being aggressive to her. Aggression can be a reaction to other factors as well—unmet physical needs, inappropriate environments, and upsetting personal interactions. A person further along in Alzheimer's might get aggressive when she feels hungry or thirsty yet is unable to identify and express those needs. Also further into the disease, unrecognized and undertreated pain can be another important and often overlooked cause of aggression. Recognizing and appropriately treating pain—a thigh bruise from bumping into a table, or an unpleasant urinary tract infection—dramatically decreases the use of psychotropic medications. Room temperature that is either too hot or too cold, a noisy environment, and lack of space for safely taking a walk are environmental stimuli that can also upset the person and lead to disturbing behaviors.

Personal interactions that do not take into account the sensibilities of the person living with Alzheimer's can also cause aggression. People may be confused when suddenly being "cared for" and consequently—and to their mind reasonably—resist attempts partners make to provide care. How would you react if someone who in your mind is a complete stranger pretended to know you and unexpectedly tried to pull down your pants? This is what the person with Alzheimer's who fights back may be experiencing. If the caring person insists on providing care at that moment, the individual may defend himself from what he sees as an unwanted approach and may even strike out because he perceives the person as an aggressor. It is important to realize that most people living with Alzheimer's do not strike out unprovoked and that partners have the responsibility to prevent what Volicer calls "resistiveness to care" from escalating into combative behavior. This can be achieved by modifying strategies for bathing, grooming, and eating, by for example, substituting washing up with a facecloth for taking a bath, delaying care until the person has calmed down, or distracting the person with stories about their past.

Damage to the orbitofrontal cortex and to the thalamus and hippocampus results in people with Alzheimer's disease having difficulty dealing with complex environmental conditions and controlling their impulses—primary symptoms of Alzheimer's disease. Finding themselves in unfamiliar and stressful social situations, they often react with anxiety, anger, or fear—all natural reactions. Unchecked feelings occasionally lead to someone hitting another person, shouting, or otherwise becoming agitated and aggressive. Damage to the brain is the physical manifestation of the disease. Loss of impulse control is a primary symptom. Feeling confused in complex social situations and acting on the feelings are secondary behaviors. Being agitated or aggressive, a natural reaction when in a questionable setting, clearly is not a disease symptom, but rather a side effect that can be alleviated.

Correctly defining and distinguishing between degrees of symptoms enables us to treat the disease and its actual symptoms more appropriately. It provides the basis for partners building new and lasting relationships. It also gives people living with Alzheimer's a better understanding of what is happening to them.

Thinking this way about primary symptoms and secondary behaviors serves as the basis for developing a truly coordinated treatment. This framework starts by acknowledging that the person living with Alzheimer's will change over time as a result of dysfunctions in the brain. Neural problems eventually lead the person to become less and less able to meet his or her own functional needs—dressing, bathing, and so on—and to getting depressed, and possibly experiencing delusions.

These direct effects in turn have side effects of their own. The person eventually becomes more dependent on others for help with daily tasks, disoriented in new places, anxious in unfamiliar situations, and unable to initiate activities that are meaningful to them.

The tertiary side effects, the next level of so-called symptoms, are really not symptoms at all, but rather reasonable reactions to external stimuli. Factors that may cause such reactions include caregiving, social environment, physical environment, and medications. Not sleeping at night, fighting with others, being agitated, refusing to eat or bathe, and being apathetic are among

SYMPTOMS, BEHAVIORS, AND SIDE EFFECTS

Primary symptoms. Clearly disease symptoms; difficulty dealing with:
- Accessing the brain's memory bank
- Accessing long-term memories without help
- Embedding new experiences into long-term memory
- Remembering where something is if it is not in view
- Remembering new spatial configurations
- Dealing with complex situations requiring sequencing and coordination
- Carrying out integrated sequences of actions
- Remaining calm in complex situations
- Finding words to express what one feels
- Keeping reality and unreality separate
- Controlling impulses when they are felt
- Keeping track of time without external cues
- Initiating meaningful activities

Secondary behaviors. Consequences that result from untreated primary symptoms.
- Inability to do certain things by oneself, such as get dressed
- Delusions
- Depression

Tertiary side effects. Behaviors that, because they are several times removed, may not actually be symptoms at all.
- Dependence on others to carry out activities of daily living including dressing, washing, eating, shaving, and so on
- Withdrawal from participating in meaningful activities
- Spatial disorientation
- Uninvoked anxiety

Nonsymptoms—falsely blaming the victim. These natural reactions of the person to the social and physical environment are not symptoms at all and may be falsely ascribed to the person as if there were no social and physical environment to which she is reacting.

Caregiving nonsymptoms
- Resistiveness leading to combativeness
- Refusing to eat, bathe, get dressed, or participate in a new activity

Social environment nonsymptoms
- Apathy
- Restlessness leading to agitation
- Repeated shouting
- Insomnia

Medical treatment nonsymptoms
- Apathy or aggression from drugs and drug interactions

Physical environment nonsymptoms
- "Escaping" from safe and controlled environments
- Interfering with other residents
- Aimless wandering

the behavioral reactions people may exhibit as a result of misalignment of these four areas with their needs.

What a coordinated treatment approach teaches us is that many behaviors that professionals and laypeople commonly refer to as Alzheimer's symptoms are not symptoms of the disease at all. As a person progresses through the disease, his brain develops certain dysfunctions. There are primary symptoms, secondary behaviors, and tertiary side effects associated with this progression, but only the primary ones caused by brain changes are actually symptoms.

As I have said, secondary behaviors and tertiary side effects are often reactions to ill-suited caregiving, social environment, medical treatment, and physical environment. Whenever I attempt to clarify these distinctions, I think about the time I injured my left-knee ligament while sitting on my knee without support in a yoga class. The primary symptom was loss of function—I could not walk as easily. When I walked more than I should have, my knee hurt—a secondary symptom. When I felt pain over a sustained period, I got irritable and nasty to people around me—a tertiary symptom. No one would define irritability and nastiness toward others as a symptom of an injured ligament, but that's what we do to people living with Alzheimer's. We blame the illness and the person for their behavior rather than looking closely at ourselves to understand what we might be doing that contributes to these outcomes.

THE FOUR A'S: APATHY, ANXIETY, AGITATION, AND AGGRESSION

Grasping what I call the four A's goes a long way to understanding Alzheimer's disease and the person living with it. If we make a mistake in how we define, categorize, respond to, and treat these four behaviors, we do more harm than good when we

THE FOUR A'S OF ALZHEIMER'S DISEASE	
Agitation—worrisome actions disruptive to others	**Anxiety**—worrying about things that can't be controlled
Aggression—striking out at others invoked by perceived aggression	**Apathy**—lack of involvement invoked by a boring environment

"help." Unfortunately, that's what most of what is called "Alzheimer's care" is doing today.

- *Agitation*—nervous behavior. The actual symptom is the lack of ability to self-initiate activities. The resulting behaviors—including restlessness, repeated actions, shouting, and talking continually—are disruptive although internally generated. Agitated behaviors are often restless responses to boredom.

- *Anxiety*—worrying about things we imagine and can't control. The actual symptom is not having a clear picture of time and causal relationships. Behaviors associated with anxiety include exhibiting nervous energy, externally communicating worry, retreating from "worrisome" social situations, and general nervousness. Something inside the person living with Alzheimer's invokes such anxiety.

- *Aggression*—striking out or shouting at others. The actual symptom is the inability to control one's own impulses.

Shouting is frequently employed, according to Jiska Cohen-Mansfield, to get the attention of others and to create something lively to take part in. Physical aggression is often an uncontrolled reaction to not understanding what is happening to one. "Why," the person asks, "am I not allowed to go out the door?"

- *Apathy*—lack of affect. The actual symptom is the inability to perceive of and remember the future, and thus the inability to plan for the future. The behavior—a response to a lack of having anything interesting to do—is nondisruptive because it is not directed at others and therefore is often not included as a symptom. A lack of stimulation in the environment invokes apathy.

IF THERE IS NO CURE, HOW CAN THERE BE A TREATMENT?

Every chronic illness faces this dilemma. AIDS, schizophrenia, and certain cancers have moved from being incurable to treatable conditions over time. AIDS was incurable and untreatable in the 1980s and 1990s; now although it is still incurable it is treatable with a mix of drugs and lifestyle changes, such as exercise, diet, and the use of condoms. In recent decades, mental illness, schizophrenia, manic depression, multiple sclerosis, and many cancers have made this shift to being treatable even though still incurable.

When dementia among the elderly was labeled "senility" and "hardening of the arteries" and was considered an attribute of natural aging, few people paid much attention to this condition because they considered it chronic, hopeless, and untreatable. Research scientist Peter Whitehouse sees the distinction between Alzheimer's brain aging and less severe brain aging as a "myth." According to Whitehouse, it's just a matter of some people's brains aging faster than others because of genetic and environmental differences. Whether you believe this or not, shifting Alzheimer's—or rapid brain aging—into the same class of illness as cancer, multiple sclerosis, diabetes, congestive heart failure, and degenerative arthritis places it squarely in the realm of an understandable and manageable condition. Making this link turns Alzheimer's into a treatable, although still incurable, condition rather than a hopeless one. This seemingly simple change can bring back to the realm of the living the tens of millions of people worldwide whom our limited thinking has condemned to a limbo in which they are merely waiting to die.

The distinction between treatment and cure can be explained with reference to my trivial yet clear example of the injury I sustained to the ligament in my knee while practicing yoga. When I forgot to support myself on a block in a seated position with my leg bent under me, my knee became hyperextended and the ligament stretched. The hyperextension became quite painful and prevented me from walking for several weeks. When I was back walking, the doctor told me to wear a knee brace for a few weeks, to ice my knee every evening, take two strong anti-inflammatory pills each morning and evening, not to reinjure it, and to have some physiotherapy when it felt better. She explained that because very little blood flowed to the ligaments, the knee would never be totally "healed" and that I should focus on strengthening the muscles above and below it to prevent future injury. My knee, I was being told, is incurable—but treatable. The treatment was a careful combination of pharmacology and nonpharmacological actions. As with Alzheimer's the underlying pathology did not disappear, but the symptoms were controlled.

Cure research is ongoing, and it's hopeful. But a cure is a long way off. Every year, billions of dollars are spent worldwide to discover a drug that can prevent the onset of Alzheimer's disease. Studies to find a cure include basic laboratory research into the body's neurology, biology, and chemistry and their interactions as they relate to the disease; animal trials to determine if applications of laboratory studies lead to the desired effects; clinical trials with randomly assigned human subjects, some of whom receive an actual drug and others a harmless placebo pill; and then multiple layers of approval by the Food and Drug Administration, at least in the United States. These procedures are thankfully in place to protect people from half-baked research and haphazard clinical experience that might be physically harmful. All these steps that are part of developing safe and effective pharmacological treatments make it unlikely that a "miracle drug" will appear on the market in the near future—at least for a decade or more—even if the root cause of the disease were discovered today.

Alzheimer's experts debate whether such studies are likely to lead to drugs that prevent the disease from taking hold, or "merely" delay its symptoms. I put "merely" in quotation marks because if a person begins to show symptoms of the disease at age eighty-five and the disease can be delayed fifteen years, the delay is as good as a cure. For those who might be susceptible to Alzheimer's late in life, if the onset is delayed beyond their life span, it will not affect them. For the 10 percent who develop symptoms earlier in life—between forty and sixty-five years of age, called early onset—the delaying strategy will help them have a longer disease-free life, but the disease will still affect them later. Because the distinction between prevention and delay is seldom made evident in discussions of Alzheimer's basic science research, it appears to many that all such research is looking for a "magic bullet" that everyone hopes is just around the corner.

Treatment means reducing symptoms and improving conditions, as well as curing illnesses.

The verb *treat* is defined in the *Cambridge Dictionary of American English* as "to do something to improve the condition of (a sick or injured person), or to try to cure (a disease), as in 'The hospital treats hundreds of patients a day,' and 'The new drug may allow us to treat diabetes more effectively.' "

The noun *treatment* is defined in the *Encarta World English Dictionary* (North American Edition) as: "provision of medical care: the application of medical care to cure disease, heal injuries, or ease symptoms"; and "medical remedy: a remedy, procedure, or technique for curing or alleviating a disease, injury, or condition as in 'a new treatment for asthma.' "

Alleviating symptoms plays a major part in "treatment" in both dictionary definitions and common parlance. Treatments for illnesses and disabilities include actions aimed at reducing related symptoms—negative side effects—of the condition. A symptom of a cold is a runny nose, of a broken leg difficulty walking, and of arthritis difficulty with fine motor skills. Actions taken to reduce runny noses, help people walk, and be able to carry out detailed tasks are treatments. AIDS, schizophrenia, bipolar disorder, and now Alzheimer's—all once considered untreatable—are presently treatable although not curable.

Treatment always includes more than just drugs. To take up again the example of a twisted and swollen knee, in addition to a painkiller, treatment includes modification to the physical environment such as a ramp or mechanical lift in extreme cases, and the use of objects including a cane or crutches, hot baths, rapidly moving water (hydrotherapy), and a knee brace.

Changes in behavior and lifestyle that reduce symptoms are also treatments. Treating a swollen knee would include avoiding rough sports, raising the leg above the hip, perhaps lying down frequently, as well as walking to rehabilitate muscles and nerves. Noncurative symptom-reducing treatment would also include prescribing pharmaceuticals such as anti-inflammatory drugs, a painkiller, or even a sleeping pill.

A mix of nonpharmacological treatments along with pharmaceutical treatments seems to be most effective in treating Alzheimer's disease and associated anxiety, depression, and cognitive loss. Clearly an approach to their coordination that employs straightforward least-cost solutions first, and more intrusive higher-cost approaches later, would be useful. "Coordinated treatment" holds the key to society's ability to deal with this growing problem.

The four A's can all be treated—that is, reduced—through a coordinated evidence-based approach in which social and physical environment as well as medications are creatively employed. The following three-part coordinated treatment approach to reducing Alzheimer's symptoms, behaviors, and side effects can be used to treat any disease or physical condition:

- *Social environment,* including communication, behavior, and activity.

- *Physical environment,* referring to the way the interior and exterior environment looks and feels.
- *Medical/pharmacological,* including treatment for excess disabilities, Alzheimer's side effects, and cognitive enhancers.

Such an approach does not imply that scientists ought to stop looking for a cure for chronic diseases such as Alzheimer's, Parkinson's, cancers of all sorts, bipolar disorder, arthritis, or lupus. But in the same vein, the search for cures ought not to prevent people suffering from these conditions from being treated to reduce their symptoms and improve their quality of life.

My own experience at Hearthstone, after over a decade of taking care of residents and responding to their needs, has shown me that the following three-step sequence works best: First, identify and assess symptoms and related behaviors. Next, apply nonpharmacological approaches. Finally, after assessing improve-

---

THREE-STEP NONPHARMACOLOGICAL AND PHARMACOLOGICAL TREATMENT APPROACH

1. Describe behavior and identify contextual triggers.
2. Adapt the caregiver, physical environment, or medication regimen—the context.
3. Employ lowest possible dosage of pharmacologic treatment to make up the difference, if needed.

---

ments, employ pharmacological interventions to reduce remaining symptoms.

A simple example of helping someone to wash himself can explain the process: A partner feels it is time to help the person living with Alzheimer's to wash up. When she tells him so—in fact she says, "Take a bath"—he resists and starts to act out at her. "It's like a prison here," he shouts. "Stop forcing me to do things I don't want to do." Instead of thinking that he is out of control, the partner looks around to figure out why he is being defensive and resistant. Then she realizes that he can't see the bathroom from where he is sitting in his lounge chair, nor does he feel dirty or think he needs a bath.

She decides to remedy the situation. She goes into the bathroom and turns on the shower so there is the sound of running water. She tells him that it has been a hard day and that she's been doing a lot of physical work. "So have you," she says. She smells under her armpits and looks away in disgust. "How do you smell?" she asks him, whiffing the air around him. Then she tells him she feels she needs to wash up a bit in the bathroom— "Listen to that shower," she says, "it really must feel good." Getting up, she fetches a washcloth and begins to wipe her own arms. "Give me your hand," she says as she gently puts the washcloth on his skin. She talks about how he used to love to take showers after coming home from work. "Remember how enjoyable it was?" she asks, and doesn't wait for an answer. After all that, if her partner goes to the bathroom she washes him a bit more with the washcloth, or if he takes off his clothes and sits in the shower on the chair she has prepared, she uses the handheld shower head to give him a shower, starting from his feet and moving up.

If his agitation and resistance continue, she contacts the doctor and asks if an antianxiety pill might calm him down enough to be a bit more agreeable with washing up the next time.

Before a symptom is treated, it must be identified, analyzed, and assessed in order to determine what to do to reduce it. Identifying a symptom means looking at its elements closely enough to understand what might be done to reduce them. To decide whether a pill is the best treatment for someone who is anxious, or whether quiet music, a hug from a friend, or getting her involved in a pastime that was formerly part of her daily life would be more effective, requires a deeper and more precise understanding of her anxiety. Observing sufficiently to identify and describe the symptomatic behavior in detail is the first step in this effort. Does she look worried, or cry out? Does she get so paralyzed with fear that she refuses to get out of bed or does she get out of bed and then worry all day long?

Determining the appropriate treatment also requires understanding the events that might have triggered the behavior. Do observations or records show that she gets more anxious around certain people or in particular places? Are there situations—like taking a trip or seeing a certain person—that make her more anxious? And what about a related illness or discomfort—an excess disability—that she can't describe, but that if treated, might reduce her anxiety. Poor eyesight and hearing loss are two frequently overlooked excess disabilities.

Once the context is understood, the caregiver, the physical environment, or medication identified as triggering the symptomatic behaviors can be modified. A nonpharmacological approach is treatment when it is applied systematically and when it measurably reduces symptoms. If nonpharmacological measures are implemented, and if conditions still remain, medication might be employed. When medications are advised they need to be applied carefully, with knowledge of their particular effects and side effects, and in as low a dosage as is required to have the desired effects.

MEDICAL TREATMENT

At present the plaques and tangles that occur in the brains of people who contract Alzheimer's disease are unavoidable. Boston researcher Nancy Emerson Lombardo suggests an antioxidant-rich diet of such foods as leafy green vegetables and blueberries. Linda Teri, a researcher in California, has demonstrated that physical exercise can reduce Alzheimer's-related depression. The popular press touts brain exercise such as daily crossword puzzles and adult education classes as anti-Alzheimer's activities. Nonetheless, it is not evident at what age living a healthy lifestyle offsets the probability of Alzheimer's. We must acknowledge how far we are from a cure as we debate the value of research and treatment options. Chemists, biologists, and neuroscientists are working feverishly to find a cure. They have the hopes of all of us with them on their quest.

In the meantime, medications are regularly employed in Alzheimer's treatment. Medical advances for treatment reported in the media generally refer to research on medications intended to enhance brain function—whether pharmacological, such as cholinesterase inhibitors, or natural, such as ginkgo biloba. Any chance that the brain can be fixed—especially by a magic pill—is greeted with great public excitement. Nevertheless, the British National Institute for Health and Clinical Excellence (NICE) recommended in 2004 that the National Health Service (NHS) no longer fund "cognitive enhancer" drugs because they provided insufficient value for the money. A barrage of complaints throughout the United Kingdom that this decision hurt people living with Alzheimer's followed from the Alzheimer's Society, the public, some politicians, and some drug companies—eventually leading to a court challenge. This very basic question clearly needs national and international public debate so that whatever resolution is reached provides the highest benefit for all.

Pills, drugs, and other medications deal with the chemistry

of the body and the brain. Many types of drugs are employed in treating Alzheimer's symptoms, among them medications for excess disability conditions, antipsychotics, antidepressants, anxiolytics, sedatives, and cognitive enhancers.

An excess disability is a secondary condition or illness that makes a primary illness appear to be more severe than it is. To return again to the strained ligament in my knee, the condition forced me to cut back on exercise for a while. Lack of exercise might have led to my gaining weight. As I slowly got heavier, the weight my knee had to carry would go up and the consequent pain would increase. More pills to relieve the pain would only have made my condition worse. The problem I actually would have had to treat was the excess disability condition that made my pain worse—my weight gain, not the pain in my knee.

Illnesses and conditions that can make the symptoms and behaviors of Alzheimer's more severe than they actually are include pneumonia and urinary tract infections (which can cause agitation), ear and sinus infections (which can cause dizziness and pain), unmonitored interaction among several medications, and uncorrected vision and hearing loss (which lead to agitation).

Antipsychotic medications are sometimes prescribed to treat hallucinations, delusions, aggression, hostility, and "uncooperativeness." Since uncooperativeness in response to anxiety among people living with Alzheimer's can easily be treated and reduced

nonpharmacologically, such as by speaking gently and explaining what is happening to the person taking into account his
point of view, it would seem well advised to apply such interventions before prescribing medications for this behavior. The
same lesson can be applied to most of the following types of
medications.

Antidepressants can also be avoided for the treatment of low
mood and irritability. Since mood improves when people with
Alzheimer's are engaged in meaningful activities in a setting with
familiar furniture and decor that they recognize, it would be pru-
dent to apply these environment and communication treatments
before using medications to control "irritability." The same is
true for anxiolytics. These medications are often drawn on to
treat anxiety, restlessness, verbally disruptive behavior, and resistance. It would make sense and would reduce the possibility of
side effects to encourage agreement in pleasant surroundings
with words that encourage reminiscence, and to employ the
drugs only if these approaches do not work.

The same responsible use of drugs is necessary for cognitive
enhancers that include and have included in the past Cognex
(tacrine), Reminyl (galantamine), Exelon (rivastigmine), Aricept
(donepezil), and Namenda (memantine). Each medication has
some side effects and is also indicated for different stages of the
disease. Research shows, for example, that donepezil is indicated

for mild/early-stage Alzheimer's, while memantine is more appropriate for late stage/advanced Alzheimer's and perhaps for a milder stage of the disease if taken with donepezil. Medications clearly are a reasonable treatment when applied after other treatments, and when applied with full understanding of their effects.

Our collective knowledge is growing by leaps and bounds about how the brain works and how much remains even with the devastation of Alzheimer's. The more we learn, the more clearly we can hear each person's special inner voice, and in turn help the person actually be there with us. If we don't do this, our very presence annihilates each person we are with who is living with Alzheimer's.

3

THE ALZHEIMER'S BRAIN

the good news and

the bad news

We take note of all the details of a disease and yet make no account of the
marvels of health.
—MARIA MONTESSORI

∞ THERE are 100 billion cells in the three-pound jellylike organ, the human brain. That's the same number of stars in our
solar system. If you look up at the sky on a clear moonless night,
you don't see a fraction of those 100 billion stars—and that's
how many cells we have in our brains. When someone dies at
the end of the course of Alzheimer's disease, his brain is likely
to have lost up to 40 percent of its weight.

That's the bad news. The good news is seldom evoked. During the twelve- to fifteen-year course of Alzheimer's, a person's
brain starts off with perhaps 90 billion cells. After a few years

this number may be reduced to 80 billion and so on. That's good news. People living with Alzheimer's still have 90 billion, or 80 billion, or 70 billion active brain cells. Those cells hold memories, the ability to learn, the ability to be creative, and to enjoy life. Alzheimer's disease damages the brain, but a lot of the brain still functions. Those cells hold hope!

Each of the 100 billion neurons in our brains has as many as 10,000 little tentacles called axons and dendrites that reach out to other cells. Tubes inside the neurons that look like railroad tracks strengthen the cells' structure, help deliver nutrients, and serve other vital functions. When people develop Alzheimer's, these tubes in certain groups of cells are affected by the tan protein and turn into balls of useless material—called tangles. At the same time, a protein called beta-amyloid starts to form clumps around and between neurons. These clumps on the outside of the neurons are called plaques. Natural, small brain cavities that hold fluids enlarge as the disease progresses and the naturally occurring folds in the brain's outer layer become more pronounced. That's the "bad news" description of the brain.

The good news is that a great deal is going on in there even as our brains get plaques, tangles, cavities, folds, and fissures.

Our brains contain hardwired, universal, preexisting images and abilities—sometimes called instincts or natural feelings. These immediately accessible abilities that help all of us to communicate in a split second with each other are equally useful in enabling people living with Alzheimer's to communicate with us and we with them. Hardwired brain capabilities have evolved over millions of years to help mankind and other animals cope with the world around us and to survive its dangers. During this evolution, some abilities and perceptions have become embedded in our genes, resulting in our being born with certain mental abilities already in place. For example, our genes contain the information that determines which of our abilities and senses develop first, and which follow at which age. We are genetically able to hear before being able to see. This is why babies still in the womb at eight months of development respond to sounds and music. And because our critical visual development begins only with the first visual exposure after birth, premature babies need to be protected from bright lights and sunshine.

The more that critical knowledge is genetically hardwired in an animal's brain, the less dependent it is on learning, and the earlier it can fend for itself. For example, because birds are hardwired for their own particular species's birdsong, they can communicate right away with siblings and parents that they are hungry or in trouble.

Researchers have discovered hardwired abilities in animals. One of the most well-known findings, associated with the work of the Nobel-laureate ethnologist Konrad Lorenz, is "imprinting"—

greylag geese think the first object they see when they break through the egg is their mother, and they follow her around as obedient goslings. This hardwired imprinting is not just to the first object they see as soon as they hatch—it is to the first *moving* object. If this subtlety were not hardwired we might expect to see lots of greylag geese standing in front of trees and bushes waiting for their "mother" to move.

Birdsong is hardwired as well. Birds of one species raised in the nest of another species of bird sing their own hardwired song as they grow to adulthood, not the song of their adoptive family. Flying south before winter is a preset skill for certain northern hemisphere migratory birds. When hatched in a planetarium with no adult birds present, these birds fly "south," or what appears to be south from the stars projected on the planetarium sky as soon as the artificial stars are set for winter. Somewhere in their genetic makeup is a stellar signal that lets them know winter is approaching. We don't know what that is, but we know it is there. Among mammals, the little vole—a mouselike creature that lives in a nest in the ground in the desert and forages by day for food and other survival needs—has hardwired traits. No matter how far desert voles roam from their burrows and no matter how circuitous the route they take in their foraging, they are born with the ability to find their way directly in a straight line back to their burrow in case of danger.

HARDWIRED HUMAN ABILITIES

Although emerging neuroscience techniques will determine with increasing precision which brain elements are hardwired in humans, we already have indications of certain hardwired human skills and memories. Among these are facial expressions, responses to the touch of another, singing, and landmarks for way-finding—all abilities that last our entire lives, even if we have Alzheimer's.

Hardwired brain functions are important for people living with Alzheimer's because they are never lost and are always accessible. New York University psychiatrist Barry Reisberg, who invented the scale to identify stages of Alzheimer's disease, has developed the evidence-based theory of Alzheimer's retrogenesis. He argues convincingly that with minor exceptions a person with Alzheimer's loses skills in inverse order to the sequence in which he or she gained them as a baby and a child. A baby develops the skill of grasping another's hand early in life. This is an instinct lost very late in the disease. Language centers develop later in childhood. These are affected earlier in the disease, and so on. Because preexisting hardwired characteristics, memories, and skills are acquired even before birth, the theory of retrogenesis would lead us to infer that these may never be lost in the brain and mind of a person living with Alzheimer's. They are always present, accessible to the person, and are therefore the building blocks for successful communication and continuing relationships.

Expressing and recognizing emotions in human facial expressions are hardwired, universal, and preexisting—they're the same in every culture. Everyone universally recognizes sadness in the face of a loved one who must leave, and the agony expressed by the face of a grief-stricken person. Anger, the expression made up of drawn-together brows, glaring eyes, and clenched teeth that lets others know that there will be trouble if whatever they are doing continues, is evident to everyone who sees it. The facial expression of surprise lasts only a few seconds, and is therefore difficult to photograph. But everyone recognizes it. Surprise often changes into fear—another hardwired emotion with a related hardwired expression: raised eyebrows and jaws open, lips stretched back. The smirk of disgust and contempt, with raised upper lip, slightly protruding lower lip, and wrinkled nose, is an expression everyone—including those living with Alzheimer's, their partners, and caregivers—recognizes easily and uses often.

There are also universal facial expressions of enjoyment. In reaction to sensory pleasure from sights, sounds, and smells, our faces express wonderment, excitement, relief, gratitude, joy, and amusement. These emotions and their expressions are evoked in those with Alzheimer's and their partners by cultural events, art experiences, and others making jokes and smiling.

Even the stories that people react to with such expressions tend to be the same. Show anyone the picture of a sad face and ask what the person has just been told. Among the first answers you will hear is: "One of his family members has just died." This is why everyone, including those with Alzheimer's, recognizes the painted-on faces of clowns as well as the stories they silently act out that make us laugh and cry.

When someone touches another, the neurotransmitter oxytocin—associated with childbirth and breast-feeding—is released in all of us, not just in women. Massage releases oxytocin as does being in homelike environments. Oxytocin is called the "care and connection" neurotransmitter because it makes us feel comfortable, open toward one another, and caring. More oxytocin is released when the front of our bodies is touched than the back, indicating that sexual contact was a root cause of this particular hardwired characteristic. Human touch is seldom misunderstood. No wonder that people living with Alzheimer's respond so well to the touch of others and to people who sincerely care for them, and are caring in return.

Babies respond to faces at certain focal distances in ways that engender bonding—much like imprinting in geese. In one experiment, two pieces of wood shaped like extended Ping-Pong paddles were shown to babies about ten inches away from their faces, the distance of a mother's face when breast-feeding. One had six lines drawn to represent a crude face—two eyes, two eyebrows, a nose, and a mouth. The other racket had the same six lines distributed haphazardly. Babies routinely responded with smiles to the more facelike racket.

My own observation of people sitting and chatting around the holographic fireplaces in each Hearthstone Residence living room has convinced me that the recognition of fire as protective is hardwired—with mental linkages to hearth, home, sociability, safety, warmth, and food.

It is likely that the need for contact with the natural environment and the feelings we have about nature and being outdoors are hardwired, partly because this is the source of our food. Sunshine, flowers, shade, moonlight, and trees are all so much a part of our basic nature that no one has to be taught to respond appropriately to such stimuli. Again not surprisingly, gardens and nature are much appreciated by those with this illness.

Babies, even fetuses after eight months, react to certain music in predictable ways. Called the Mozart effect, because the effect of Mozart's music on babies has been studied extensively, it appears that music with predominantly higher pitch has this effect more than other music. Although the precise reasons for this are not clear, it is certain that responding to and making music are hardwired. Recent research indicates that song— narrative music expressing strong emotions, even without explicit words—is likely to have predated language as a form of communication.

Understanding how much innate knowledge and experience there is to mine in the brain can help everyone interacting with those living with Alzheimer's to communicate, plan supportive environments, and maintain and establish healthy and healing relationships.

THE ALZHEIMER'S BRAIN IS A CREATIVE BRAIN

Three major brain functions, each representing one dimension of creativity, constitute the brain's creative process. Understanding how these three brain operations work together, and which function better and less well in Alzheimer's disease, provides a window into the brain that enables everyone, including people living with Alzheimer's, to further develop and improve their social relationships.

The three parts are:

- *The Interpreter:* Located in the left brain, the interpreter enables us to make sense of the world around us by developing images of reality, stories that interpret what we sense, and generally providing a holistic vision of the world and our relationship to it. Such images can be about the past and the present, and they can be images of the future as part of plans of action. The interpreter is always at work whenever we make sense of new and complex situations or just cope with daily life. This part of the brain functions well in people living with Alzheimer's disease, who can make up stories as well as anyone else.

• *The Actor:* The chameleonlike "actor" moves around the brain depending on the stage of perception and action being engaged in. Based on the interpreter's images, the brain perceives, conceptualizes, and engages the rest of our body to act on the picture we develop of ourselves and of the world around us. People living with Alzheimer's disease maintain their internal actors as do others their age, but they are less aware of the limitations their bodies and minds put on them. For example, throughout the illness, people living with Alzheimer's whose cognitive mapping ability is impaired still are happy to walk away from home without realizing they may get lost if they walk on a public street.

• *The Comparer:* Without even being aware, people continually assess the outcomes of their actions by comparing what actually happens to what they expected would happen. If we dress for warm weather and find that it is colder outside than we thought, we return home to add another layer of clothing. If we expect to find our car parked on the third level of the garage and it isn't there, we try another floor. On the basis of such comparisons taking place in our brains, we revise our images of reality.

The brain's comparer is located in the A-10 nucleus of the frontal lobe with a connection to the occipital lobe. The comparer in the brain of a person living with Alzheimer's disease is damaged early in the illness and continues to work less and less well throughout the Alzheimer's journey. When this happens he may repeat an action over and over even when the results are not what he wanted. For example, he might repeatedly try to open a door that is clearly locked, or stand up to walk when it is evident to others that he is unsteady on his feet. To continue functioning as well as possible, the person living with Alzheimer's needs to replace the brain's damaged comparer with visual aids, signs, helpers, and other ways to correct himself.

Understanding these three brain functions enables everyone to better comprehend and therefore communicate. For example, if a person with Alzheimer's living alone or with a partner fills his day with tasks and adventures that rely primarily on the interpreter in the brain, he is likely to have a successful day full of quality experiences. Farther into the disease, activities that stimulate the brain's "actor" functions, such as museum visits, short films, and listening to poetry, are extremely accessible to people living with Alzheimer's. While it is always good to exercise our brains, activities that rely primarily on the person's brain comparer—his ability to review what has happened and to revise a perception or expressed attitude—are likely to be more difficult and lead to greater frustration. These include any task that requires comparison of a recent experience with an experience of the past—comparing today's weather or movie to yesterday's weather or movie, for example.

The more we understand the brain—its hardwired capabilities and its creative capacities—the better we can organize activities and communicate with each other during the passage of Alzheimer's. At the same time we have to dispel several overly simplistic and therefore easily adopted myths related to the Alzheimer's brain.

THE MYTH OF SHORT-TERM AND LONG-TERM MEMORY

Alzheimer's disease is popularly seen as memory loss because on the surface a person appears to "forget" things—a message she was supposed to pass on, a name, or an appointment. This occurs because the hippocampus—a key part of the brain that is crucial to indexing experiences, to inserting them into long-term memory, and to retrieving all memories—is damaged early in the progress of the illness. Because hippocampal damage results in people not being able to index and insert experiences into their brains as easily as before, it appears to others that the person is having difficulty remembering immediate experiences soon after they occur. Most people believe that the main symptom associated with Alzheimer's is that people "forget" things, but it is not.

The degree of difficulty a person has indexing and then re-calling an event changes throughout the illness—with there be-ing less and less ability over time. The oversimplified view that people living with Alzheimer's lose their short-term memory while keeping their long-term memory is not helpful in under-standing the full complexity of the person, nor does it lead to developing effective treatment or to living a quality life.

This one-dimensional view leads to treatments that are di-rected toward memory alone, when the cognitive and neuro-science picture of the person living with Alzheimer's is more dynamic and deserves a less crude approach. The person is also more complex and dynamic and deserves to be treated with greater interest, understanding, and respect. While a significant player in the Alzheimer's brain is the hippocampus—making what appears to be "memory loss" a major factor—a fuller ex-position of the Alzheimer's brain provides a richer multidimen-sional picture, leading to more fine-tuned treatments.

The hippocampus is the key to the brain's memory bank—just as your car key unlocks the glove compartment where maps and other information are stored. The hippocampus is a small sea horse–shaped organ in the brain's limbic system, a set of structures that supports a variety of functions including emotion and long-term memory. It provides each of us access to the memories we have already stored. Neuroscientist Bruce Mc-Naughton at the University of Arizona describes the hippocampus as "indexing each experience and thus memory for later recall." The hippocampus enables us to embed new memories, including thoughts and feelings about new experiences, into our long-term memory banks, tagging them for later retrieval. Because this brain element is damaged early in the illness, people seem to have difficulty "remembering" things that have just happened, and even things that happened long ago—unless they are prompted and cued by a person or object in their context. As with Marcel Proust in *In Search of Lost Time*—whose memories were awakened by the taste of a madeleine at his grandmother's house—tastes, smells, and visual images enhance access to memories for people living with Alzheimer's.

All of our many memories are in our brains. We don't forget our children, our joys and sorrows, or our relationships that easily. It is just harder to access them without help.

If you have gone through a traumatic experience or even have come home very drunk one night, you know what this feeling is like. You know you have had an experience but, for the life of you, you can't place a particular phrase or person in the memory of the experience. Once someone prompts you with a fact or a picture, things begin to come into focus. That's what it is like to have a damaged hippocampus. It is not surprising that cueing memories with key words, photos, and music is a tried-and-true method of therapeutic interaction with people who are living with Alzheimer's. Knowing this, people recently diagnosed with Alzheimer's can help themselves by establishing supportive cuing systems before they are needed.

My colleague Cameron Camp has developed an exciting research-based approach to Alzheimer's treatment by demonstrating that people living with Alzheimer's can definitely learn and remember new things when taught systematically, slowly, and in precise and expanding time intervals. Called "spaced retrieval," this technique employs procedural learning—the way we learn to ride a bike, drive a car, and use chopsticks—to patiently guide people living with Alzheimer's to embed new memories in their brains. Using repetition and repeated success, people living with Alzheimer's can learn and can remember. In public presentation, Cameron quickly gets any audience to realize that people living with Alzheimer's can learn at every stage of the illness. He asks the audience of caregivers, "What happens when you seat someone else in Mary's chair in the dining room at lunchtime?" When members of the audience reply, "Mary gets angry or upset," Cameron points out that before moving to the residence, Mary didn't know where her chair was. She must have learned it since getting there. How did she do this?

Damage to the executive function area in the frontal lobe makes it difficult for people living with Alzheimer's to organize sequences of events into a single process. This occurs early in the progress of Alzheimer's for most people, although like other characteristics, this challenge increases over time. Someone living with Alzheimer's doesn't "forget" how to get dressed or brush his teeth; it is just more difficult to put all the steps in the right order for such multistage activities. Getting dressed, for example, requires finding the closet and dresser, knowing where various items of clothing are stored, selecting the right items of clothing for the weather and activities of the day, selecting items of clothing coordinated to each other, taking out all the items and arranging each front to front and outside out, putting them on in the correct order, and finally zipping, buttoning, and fastening. Over fifty steps are required just to get dressed, and that's only one of the sequences we need to perform every day. Brushing teeth, taking a shower, cooking breakfast, traveling to work, driving a car, paying bills, and shopping are all extremely complex sequences. Most people carry out these activities of daily living easily and automatically without being conscious of the complexity of the tasks they are doing with so little effort or the difficulty others might have with the same tasks.

People living with Alzheimer's with damaged frontal lobe executive function find it difficult to carry out seemingly simple operations that are actually extremely complex sequences. While the person appears to increasingly "forget" how to do these things, it's not a memory problem. If the props for the task are appropriately set up and visible—the toothpaste, the water glass, and the toothbrush, or the appropriate sequence of clothing with which to get dressed, people living with Alzheimer's tend to "remember" what needs to be done with the props, and they can complete the tasks successfully.

Other brain organs are involved with impulse control—stopping us from acting impulsively even when we feel like it. When you or I get angry with someone in a social setting we do not immediately punch him. If we feel sexually attracted to someone else in public we do not immediately expose ourselves or touch the other person inappropriately. Most of the time when we feel angry and do something we later regret, we admonish ourselves to better control our actions rather than believe we should not have felt the anger in the first place. A healthy orbitofrontal cortex, thalamus, and hippocampus serve as inhibitors to potentially destructive behaviors. As these organs are damaged more and more during the progress of Alzheimer's, the person increasingly "acts out" the way he feels—the way we might under great stress. This lack of social impulse control is not "forgetting" how to behave; it is losing control over naturally occurring feelings. Organizing social events and physical environments that elicit appropriate behaviors is one way to avoid inappropriate social behaviors in someone with less impulse control. This can be done simply. For example, if someone tends to get angry easily, make sure that a birthday party thrown for him, is held in a dining room rather than an institutional community room, that he sits next to a favorite grandchild toward whom he feels protective, and that the grandchild wears a festive name tag with her first name in large letters. The dining room lets him know "dinner behavior" is appropriate, the grandchild evokes hardwired caring instincts, and the name tag cues his memory.

HALLUCINATIONS AND DELUSIONS

Someone living with Alzheimer's or another dementia may at times feel that something has occurred that hasn't, or that someone or something is present that isn't. My friend and mentor Paul Raia, director of patient care and family support at the Massachusetts Alzheimer's Association, sees people with Alzheimer's and family members who are living with difficult situations such as these. Among the stories he hears from time to time are:

- Looking directly at his wife, a man says, "You're not my wife. You look like her, but you're not her."
- Seeing shadows on the wall from a streetlight outside a window, a woman comes out of her room frightened and says, "There's someone lurking in my room."
- Seeing several people in her home whom she does not recognize, a sociable woman complains, "I didn't invite these people to my party, and I can't afford to feed them all. Tell them to go home."

- When the mail arrives, a man who has difficulty handling bills gets angry because "people keep writing me strange letters."

In the case of the misperceived wife, the damaged system is emotional. The person sees and recognizes his wife (visual and perceptual systems), but something emotional just doesn't compute. He doesn't feel about her as he knows he would feel if the person were his wife. The second is an example of a damaged visual and perceptual system—the shifting shadows look like a person hiding in the shadows. The third is psychologically based: the person feels that everyone she sees is taking advantage of her generosity. The last is an example of paranoia.

The first line of attack in these and similar situations is to ask, "Why is this happening?" If the problem is emotional or visual, changing the context might help. For example, the woman who is not recognized by her husband might quietly leave the room, then reenter smiling broadly and saying, "Hi, Joshua, I'm your wife, Sylvia, and we love each other very much." If her husband says that someone very similar was just there, Sylvia might respond that perhaps the person who was there was one of the many people who look just like her. If moving shadows are causing a problem, someone can close the curtains at night and turn on a soft light.

Psychological and paranoid hallucinations and delusions are

more difficult to affect nonpharmacologically and might require more immediate medical interventions. Researchers studying such matters have identified paranoid or misidentification delusions, such as thinking that a spouse is an imposter and that the house is not home, and "factual delusions" such as believing that one is the director of a program when one is actually a participant. Some factual mistakes are the result of poor memory and eyesight, and should not be mistaken for delusions.

Delusions such as these result in part from damage to the brain's comparer. If the comparer in the frontal lobe is damaged, the person has greater difficulty monitoring what is real, comparing internal experience with external "facts," linking new experiences with memories of the past, and preventing the person from consolidating inaccurate beliefs in the brain.

Knowing that delusions and hallucinations are a result of specific brain changes ought to help partners realize that the person living with Alzheimer's is not "crazy." It also enables them to accept that in many cases a specific action can help reduce hallucinations and delusions, such as leaving the room and reintroducing oneself, showing the person his or her professional diploma, or changing the lighting or the window shades to get rid of shadows.

When the person you have lived with for fifty years says you are not yourself, or that the house he is living in isn't his, it can be frightening. Sometimes, however, delusions provide valuable insights into the person's inner emotional needs that can give partners direction as to how best to help the person. For example, someone whose paranoia directs her to accuse her daughter of taking her handbag might be letting others know she feels that her personal identity is missing. After all, what is kept in a handbag except one's "personal identity," and if you don't have your bag how do you know who you are? All your important stuff is in that bag. That particular delusion tells us that what may be needed to make her whole is to give her purpose and make her feel like a person who is valued. Delusions and hallucinations, as Freud thought, can be road maps to the psyche—albeit in this example, a psyche distorted by disease.

Not all delusions and hallucinations are bad things that need to be changed. But when they cause the person constant pain, or are dangerous to the person or others, and can't be changed non-pharmacologically, medications are likely to be needed.

LANGUAGE

Wernicke's area and Broca's area in the brain, named after the physiologist and neurologist who discovered them, control our understanding of words we hear and our ability to recall words that express what we mean to say—receptive and expressive spoken language. Language centers become impaired more in the middle of the disease than in the early period and more among some people than others. When this happens those people may be less able to find the words they need to express themselves or they appear not to be able to understand others. These two deficits do not necessarily go hand in hand. A person with temporal-lobe dementia is likely to have greater difficulty in finding the words to express a thought than in understanding others.

Just because a person living with Alzheimer's is not able to find certain words, she is likely to know the meaning of what she wants to say—somewhere deep inside she knows what she wants to say. The trick in the relationship is to use all the other senses we have to read what the other person is trying to express— touch, "I love you," "You must be feeling sad," and a hug—and to divine the implicit meaning in a situation.

OUR SENSE OF TIME

When an area called the chiasmatic nucleus is damaged, our natural internal time clock—set closer to a twenty-five-hour day than twenty-four hours—goes haywire. Our internal clock enables us to know what time of day it is even if we are closeted in a windowless conference room for hours. Someone living with Alzheimer's is likely to have difficulty doing this; he might think it is the middle of the night because he has not seen daylight for as long as he can remember. This leads, among other things, to his asking repeatedly, "When are we leaving?" or waking up in the middle of the night thinking that it's daytime, or feeling anxious when the end of the day is evident—a phenomenon known as *sundowning.*

"Zeitgebers"—time-givers in the environment—remind us of the correct time and help us orient ourselves to time throughout the day. The sun and the weather are excellent zeitgebers because they naturally align people's internal clocks. Someone recently diagnosed with Alzheimer's who wants to avoid temporal dislocation should take walks outside regularly to set their clocks. One hour in sunshine every morning is the best zeitgeber. Residential group settings for people living with Alzheimer's, such as special assisted-living programs for those with cognitive problems, often include access to a garden designed for safety, way-finding, and place awareness. Walking in such a specially planned treatment or healing garden as a way to reset the body's clock is an important treatment for sleep-wake and other temporal disturbances.

EMOTION

Located in the limbic system near the hippocampus, the amygdala maintains its function late into the disease and is the key to communicating and having a fulfilling relationship with a person living with Alzheimer's. Whenever we have an emotional reaction to a person, event, or place, or we express ourselves emotionally, our amygdalas are at work. This almond-shaped organ (*amygdale* is the word for "almond" in Greek) processes our emotions in our brains—particularly emotions of anger and hate—but also love and caring. The amygdala is healthy far into the disease, making people with Alzheimer's exquisitely sensitive to emotional events and other people's emotional states. Partners who connect on an emotional level—reading each other's emotions and expressing themselves emotionally—can communicate effectively even if one is living with Alzheimer's.

In sum, a great deal more goes on in the brain of a person living with Alzheimer's than mere memory loss. We need to be sensitive to all the changes if we are to avoid throwing out the baby with the bathwater—if we are not to discard the person merely because we can't deal with a "loss of memory."

4

ART AND ALZHEIMER'S

how to connect with
someone through
visual art

Art reveals to us the essence of things, the essence of our existence.

—RUDOLF ARNHEIM

∞ VISITING ART MUSEUMS and attending poetry readings and concerts are relaxing diversions in a life focused on family, work, and even recreation. Few of us integrate artistic expression into our daily lives, or even attend performances and art exhibits regularly. Professional artists are the exception. We are the poorer for it. We each have a need and natural aptitude for art that we realize how much we miss only when we find ourselves without other supports in our lives.

For older people in general and people living with Alzheimer's disease in particular who have lost work roles and take part in fewer intimate family activities, engagement in art and art experiences play a special role. The arts can provide meaning in what to many is experienced as an ever increasingly meaningless life. Art connects people to their culture and to their community. It gives meaning to life and it is meaning that people living with Alzheimer's so dearly crave.

Alzheimer's brings with it added sensitivity and openness to art, even for someone who may have had little artistic aptitude in the past. The person realizes this through taking part in art experiences. In order for these effects to take place, partners also have to believe that the person they love who is living with Alzheimer's without a strong short-term memory can actually have satisfying and enriching art experiences.

Art may be therapeutic, but doing art isn't necessarily therapy. When you play with your dog at home, it is not pet therapy. When you plant or harvest vegetables in your garden, it is not horticultural therapy. When you entertain your grandchildren and their friends, it is not intergenerational therapy. Similarly, when you paint a serious picture or visit an art gallery as a hobby or for fun, it is not art therapy, although it may have therapeutic effects. Why do we label such activities as therapy when people living with Alzheimer's engage in them? Because we do not really believe people with this disease can truly enjoy such an experience as we do, we doubt they remember it, and therefore we do not encourage art experiences as an integral part of their everyday lives.

When art is a profound part of the everyday flow of life for people living with Alzheimer's, it offers a vibrant and extraordinary dimension.

Art touches and engages the brain in a more profound way than other activities. Music, painting, sculpture, comedy, drama, poetry, and the other arts link together separate brain locations in which memories and skills lie. The brain systems affected in this way are therefore called "distributed." Music, for example, touches parts of the brain that link what we sense, know, and feel. As the brain is affected in Alzheimer's disease and particular locations and abilities are damaged, the fact that art touches so many areas of the brain masks single-location deficits.

The more someone is in touch with his or her feelings, the more he or she can appreciate art. The same is true for creating art. Artists who think too much edit their works mentally before they can express them. Because people living with Alzheimer's tend to express what they think and feel at the moment, they are natural artists and natural audiences for artistic expression.

Various arts are also hardwired in the brain. We know that a fetus late in its development responds to music. A young child does not have to be taught to relax when she hears a lullaby, nor does she need to be taught to paint colorful pictures, or to laugh at a silly joke. These universal, preexisting, and hard-wired abilities, lost only late in the progress of Alzheimer's if at all, serve as the basis for successful art expression and appreciation throughout the progress of the disease.

With my friend and colleague Sean Caulfield, I founded Artists for Alzheimer's (ARTZ), a program that accesses all these attributes of art and art experience for people living with Alzheimer's. The program, as I'll explain it here, can serve as a model for individuals to connect with cultural events in their own communities.

The following description of the ARTZ program is relevant to everyone living with Alzheimer's and their partners. Each person and every partner can look for and take advantage of such programs in their own community and use the principles presented here to assess their quality. If art programs don't exist, people can ask that such a program be initiated, and can even work at setting one up themselves. And of course, as I shall describe at the end of this chapter, each person can use the principles of visual art experience at home as part of the relationship being developed.

ARTZ asks creative people, both professional performers and regular folks who just like to sing, to volunteer for a specific amount of time each year. The time requested cannot be refused—one hour per year. ARTZ volunteers spend their hour either performing for an audience or leading a hands-on workshop with people living with Alzheimer's. During this one hour participants enjoy themselves, feel successful, and possibly discover talents they did not know they had. Volunteer artists who find out what a wonderful audience and group of participants people living with Alzheimer's are tell others, and the message spreads, reducing the stigma still further. Many return over and over. The "regulars" who integrate these art exchanges into their daily lives at least once a month become ARTZ artists in residence.

Tanya Azarani, the first ARTZ artist in residence, conducted a series of art classes with residents over several months. She began by teaching technique, employing watercolor, acrylic paint, and colored pencil. Then she moved on to conduct several classes concerned with still life drawing and copying photographs, to give participants a sense of creating an art object. She ended by getting participants to use art to express who they are—to express their "selves" through art. This is something you can do with your partner if you are inclined to the visual arts.

The program's aim is twofold. First, ARTZ provides people living with Alzheimer's with regular artistic experiences—performances and hands-on involvement by competent artists of all ages. Artists include comedians performing stand-up comedy, actors reading plays and poetry, photographers taking pictures and sharing their work, industrial designers and sculptors working in clay, guitarists and violinists performing, painters and graphic artists, and opera singers.

The program's second aim is to enable artists to experience the joy of working with and performing for people living with Alzheimer's. Many of the performers have or have had family members living with the disease and find ARTZ a way for them to give back to that community. For others, this is the first time they have interacted with people living with Alzheimer's. After their own "art experiences" with residents, the artists become ambassadors to the larger world, spreading the message that people living with Alzheimer's are "people" first, not just persons with a disease.

The results of Tanya's art classes were extraordinary. People who had never painted before expressed themselves eloquently through art. Just one example of this was former New York City policeman Frank Ertola, whose watercolor still life *Iris* is an elegant and sensitive artwork.

The classes also produced a vivid painting of a bear. Wolf Goldstein, a ninety-five-year-old concentration camp survivor, painted the bear and signed the painting with his first name—resulting in a mistaken-identity title on the upper right-hand corner of the painting. Why is this important for people living with Alzheimer's and their families? An example of the significance lies in the reaction of Wolf's son to one of his father's paintings. Wolf did not speak a great deal, yet he eloquently and profoundly expressed himself in his "Who am I?" painting—its repeated vertical lines seeming to express "prison," and a six-pointed star representing his religious identity. When his son saw the painting, he was moved to learn that so much feeling was still alive in his father. You too can achieve contact with your partner's feelings through art communication.

For each person coping with Alzheimer's, living in a world with less stigma associated with the condition will ease their burden. To achieve the goal of destigmatizing Alzheimer's it is essential that the art people living with Alzheimer's create be respectfully shared with the general public. In 2004, the John Michael Kohler Art Center in Sheboygan, Wisconsin, and patron Mark Nemschoff decided to sponsor a traveling exhibition of fifty-one ARTZ program paintings and drawings that Tanya's students created. The exhibition has since been hosted at Banner Health Foundation in Phoenix, at the Massachusetts Alzheimer's Association offices, in the lobby of a laboratory of a major pharmaceutical company in Boston that has no Alzheimer's drug on the market, and in Boston's Jordan Hall at a Longwood Symphony Orchestra concert.

Like other companies, this one has scientists researching the illness. But unlike other companies, the head of the laboratory wanted scientists there to reach through Alzheimer's to see the people for whom they are working. He decided to exhibit the paintings so that researchers could see and realize that those people are "still there."

The Kohler Art Center is a major exhibition and performance center for "outsider art"—art by artists who have little or no professional training—and this is how the art was presented. The fifty-one pieces constituted an outsider art exhibition, not the art output of people with an illness. The audience at the Kohler Art Center consisted of adults and children interested in artistic expression of all sorts.

At the Banner Health Foundation the audience included health care professionals as well as people coming to the hospital for health care. Pam O'Neil, a registered nurse on the staff at the hospital, expresses the impact this artistic expression had on her:

I was moved by the feelings that washed over me, I could feel the artists' energies coming off the pieces. They are in there!!!! and how wonderful to communicate in this way—no misunderstandings—right here right now, their feelings. And I was moved to know that this would not be a lost memory. I could share and their families could share and the community could share and see that these people are real, and a real moment in time was recorded for them. Because of this, I am sure that the art from our patients and our community belongs on our hospital's walls.

Most ARTZ participants are individuals, but not all. A growing number of creative organizations have joined the Artists for Alzheimer's program as members and together with ARTZ they have partnered to develop exciting joint programs. Organiza-

tions include the Bowery Poetry Club together with the Santa
Fe Alzheimer's Poetry Project, the Tribeca Film Institute, New
York's Big Apple Circus, the Spruill Art Center in Atlanta, the
Cirque Phénix, in Paris, organizers of the Circus Festival of
Tomorrow, the Harvard Museum of Natural History, and the
National Heritage Museum in Lexington, Massachusetts. One
dream I have is to see cultural institutions in every major world
city open their doors and develop programs for people with
Alzheimer's—Sydney, London, Paris, Seoul, Florence, Madrid,
San Francisco, as a start. There is no reason that every major cul-
tural organization in the world should not open its arms regu-
larly to this group of vibrant and alive people.

MUSEUM TOURS

To broaden the range of meaningful art experiences available to
people living with Alzheimer's, ARTZ develops guided tours for
them worldwide. Among the first such programs ARTZ developed was at the Louvre in Paris, at the National Gallery of Australia in Canberra, and at the Museum of Modern Art (MoMA)
in New York City. At the Louvre, Cindy Barotte, who pio-
neered ARTZ in France, guides visitors with Alzheimer's and
their partners through the French, Flemish, and Italian Renais-
sance galleries on Tuesdays, when the Louvre is closed to the
general public. At MoMA, the tours are also conducted on

Tuesdays, when the museum is closed to the public, so that there is minimal distraction. ARTZ creative director Sean Caulfield devised the title "Meet Me at (the Museum) . . . and Make Memories" for this program—an active and creative name and objective. Tours in these museums as well as museums throughout the Boston area and elsewhere promise an Alzheimer's-friendly environment and Alzheimer's-capable trained educators leading the discussions of the paintings and sculpture specially selected for this population.

At museums that have such programs, anyone who wants to can call the museum to reserve a place in the next set of tours—several are conducted simultaneously so that the size of each group is kept to about five or six participants with one educator. Each participant comes alone if they are able, or brings a partner of their choice. At a recent MoMA tour I observed, all the participants were women, although men often attend as well. One came by herself, another was accompanied by three of her grandchildren, another by her husband, and one talkative and insightful woman who had been there before and clearly plans to be part of every tour she can, came with her aide. One important action you can take with your partner is to take advantage of such programs where they do exist and advocate for at museums you frequent without such tours.

ARTZ initially piloted a community-oriented program with MoMA in which groups of people with Alzheimer's living together in assisted-living or nursing homes participated in a three-part program. First a museum educator visits the residence and leads a discussion, projecting art images on a screen and handing out large-postcard-size reproductions of selected museum artwork to residents. Residents are left with these reproductions of the artworks to hang, review, and enjoy before they visit the museum. A guided museum visit where the same artworks are on display and discussed is the second step. The tour ends with participants making drawings of one of the paintings in the gallery; once when I was there the painting selected was Matisse's *Dancing Nudes* hanging high on the wall in a large well-lit lobby area, out of the way of any traffic there might be. Participants were given a white card attached to a small clipboard and asked to draw what they saw. The results were remarkable. One participant with advanced Alzheimer's drew an exquisite stick figure that exceptionally expressed the emotion and rhythm of one of the dancers. You too can do this with a partner at a local museum.

In the third part of this program, educators return to the residence where participants make drawings of the art using colored pencil and pipe cleaners. This last session begins with each participant bringing to the table and telling stories about an object from their lives that is personally significant for him or her. Family photographs, jewelry, and antiques are discussed, inviting the full person to the table and building bridges between members of the group.

Museum educators are trained to engage people of all ages and backgrounds in art. Skilled educators know how to present art and to elicit participants' responses and opinions to specific artworks. They know how to make everyone's opinion count, and to provide just enough information so that viewers feel they have learned something without being overwhelmed. In order to engage people living with Alzheimer's in such art discussions, they need special training first to choose paintings that elicit the cognitive strengths of participants, and then to employ a question-asking approach that elicits participants' perception and discussion.

At local museums, ARTZ staff members develop programs by first interviewing people living with Alzheimer's about their reactions to an array of paintings, sculptures, and photographs at the museum. At the Louvre, initial interviews to select paintings for the tour were conducted for people living with Alzheimer's at the long-term-care Bretonneau hospital. Images to test in this way were selected from those available on the Louvre website in the physical area we had decided to visit. At MoMA, ARTZ staff used as the basis for its artwork selection research a boxed set of thirty reproductions called "MoMA in a Box." The artwork selection in each museum begins with focused interviews with people who have Alzheimer's, who are presented with reproductions. They—not the educators, the museum, or even ARTZ staff—select the art to be included in the tour.

The standardized focused interview question used in this selection phase to elicit responses is: "I want to buy some paintings
to hang on the wall of the hallway here, and I need some advice.
Could you please look at these pictures and tell me whether you
think I should buy the artwork to hang it up here?" If such a
methodology is not used, the tours run the risk of becoming the
reflection of tour guides' image of what a person living with
Alzheimer's can handle, rather than the reality of the condition.
At MoMA, where ARTZ piloted the first of its many museum
tours, thirty prints were presented to respondents in the selection
interviews. Ten paintings seemed to be totally not understandable, ten other prints were understood by some and not by others, and ten everyone understood. Of the ten well-understood
artworks, participants considered five to be too risqué to hang up
in a home while five were more than acceptable.

When experts are asked to rate the way they believe participants evaluated the prints, they are usually half wrong. This is
what happened the first time the MoMA docents tried to guess
the answers ARTZ staff found among its respondents living
with Alzheimer's, and the same tends to be the case in other
groups of museum educators as well. Getting inside the minds
of people living with Alzheimer's requires more than intuition.

Artworks that the data indicate people living with Alzheimer's best understand tend to evoke six particular reactions.
Participants indicate their understanding by describing clearly

and openly what they see, interpreting the story of the painting, seeing in it some link to their own lives, expressing the emotion of the artwork, identifying objects, and critically appraising the subject matter. You can use these same criteria to guide you in your own museum visits with family members.

People living with Alzheimer's understand visual art by:

1. *Perceiving and describing*—talking about what they see in the artwork.
2. *Telling a story*—narrating the story they see in the painting.
3. *Linking it to their own lives*—describing personal and historical memories.
4. *Identifying the emotion*—naming and expressing the emotions in the artwork.
5. *Identifying objects that make up the painting*—seeing, naming, and describing the objects.
6. *Making critical judgments*—commenting on moral issues raised in "risqué" artwork.

In the initial ARTZ tours at MoMA, discussion of paintings and sculpture focused on artworks selected from the ten "understood" artworks, as well as several from the "partly understood" group. These latter paintings engage the curiosity of participants and engender lively conversation when the exceptional guides point out and explain characteristics of each painting and engage participants through insightful questioning. During some tours, docents were encouraged to test a new painting in the exhibition with participants, but to carefully observe if the new painting was clearly understood or not.

On the basis of its research, ARTZ recommended that seven paintings serve as the focus of most tours.

Wyeth's *Christina's World* was the most easily understood painting. Many people know it well. A woman sits at the lower left corner of the painting, in a field of yellow-green grass, looking at a farmhouse in the upper right corner. You see only the back of her body in the grass, but you know there is a connection between her and the farmhouse. Here's what research subjects said: "There is something special about that house." "She is yearning for something in the house." "She wants to get to the house. So do I."

The actual story of Christina is that she had been physically disabled by a childhood attack of polio, and was able to move around the property only by pulling herself along with her arms and hands. Interestingly, participants with Alzheimer's are so attuned to what Wyeth expressed in the painting that they generally notice that Christina has physical problems just from observing the painting itself, with no further explanation. A quite amazing thing occurred on one visit. Reuben Rosen, a tour participant with some art experience, said critically: "Her arms and legs are spindly, but she has a really healthy butt, and that's a mistake." When Reuben made that observation, I immediately saw what he saw in the painting, and have seen it ever since—but I had no explanation for why such an accomplished painter would have made such a "mistake." Recently I found out why.

At a flea market on Martha's Vineyard last summer, I bought a used book of essays on and interviews with Wyeth. In one of the interviews he explains that he was embarrassed to ask Christina to model for the painting: "Finally I got up enough courage to say to her, 'Would you mind if I made a drawing of you sitting outside?' and drew her crippled arms and hands. . . . I was so shy about posing her, I got my wife Betsy to pose for her figure." Reuben was right.

Few respondents "understood" Mondrian's *Broadway Boogie Woogie,* a large canvas with colorful rectangles arranged in straight horizontal and vertical lines. Most said things like "Why would someone want to hang a tablecloth on the wall?" But when a docent gave them the title, their minds quickly jumped to Times Square and dancing the boogie-woogie in dance clubs when they were young. They remarked that the colors in the Mondrian reminded them of Broadway.

Museum tours do not just "happen," and museums that do not follow all the steps to guarantee that their tours will be

Alzheimer's-competent run the risk of having a negative effect on people and their partners. Museum educators who carry our Alzheimer's tours, in addition to learning basic techniques for dealing with groups of any age relating to art, must also learn how to relate to people living with Alzheimer's. This latter training includes specific tips on helping participants in the museum to feel comfortable in this new situation. Training sessions include discussion of artworks that research has shown resonate with people living with Alzheimer's, demonstrations, and supervised tours with potential clients, followed by discussion and critique. Artwork selection and tour guide training principles apply to all the museums at which ARTZ has made such tours available, including the Louvre, the Harvard University Museum of Natural History, MoMA, the DeCordova Museum & Sculpture Park in Lincoln, Massachusetts, and many others. You can use the same principles when you visit museums yourself with your partner, and when you set up guided museum visits.

Here are the Artists for Alzheimer's museum program communication principles:

- *Scope out the building.* Map the building. Plan how participants will get around the building so that their experience is most enjoyable and least jarring.

- *Set the stage.* Prework. Have name tags ready for participants. Decide on using first or last names in addressing participants. Ask, "Would you like me to call you Mary or Mrs. Smith?"

- *Introduce yourself.* Wear your name tag. Point to your first name when you introduce yourself. Identify yourself by name; explain simply what your role is.

- *Employ friendly body language.* Stand in front of the person, to be least threatening. Hold their hand. Look into their eyes. Smile.

- *Alleviate participants' anxiety about where they are.* Answer the question "Where are we?" without being asked. Repeat regularly, "We are at the Central City Museum here in Minneapolis," or whatever city you are in.

- *Alleviate participants' anxiety about why they are there.* Answer the question "Why are we here?" without being asked. Repeat as often as necessary, "We will be looking at wonderful works of art." (What do they want me to do?) "Your family and friends know that you are here." (What if my wife is looking for me!) "We will be here for one hour." (When am I leaving?)

- *Involve each participant.* Frame the question: Relate the question to something specific in the work. For instance, "Why is that woman standing there?" Not, "What does this represent to you?" The second question will be answered in the response to the first question.

- *Avoid testing.* Don't say, "Who painted this, do you know? Come on, this one is real easy!" Instead, slowly reveal the work of art with simple descriptions and questions, thereby allowing participants to explore the artwork with you. In this way they maintain their dignity and sense of accomplishment.

- *Make the experience positive.* Positive experiences lead to self-esteem and self-esteem lasts a long time as an Alzheimer's treatment, reducing agitation, aggression, and social withdrawal. If you see someone getting anxious, change the subject.
- *Positively reinforce.* When they "get it," or get a painter's name or anything about the artwork, be positive without seeming surprised.
- *Make everything failure free.* The entire experience is supposed to be failure free—to touch their amygdala, the emotion center of the brain—positively. Don't ask participants to compare paintings they saw half an hour earlier with the one they are looking at.

After presenting these principles, the local educators at the National Gallery in Canberra, Australia, introduced me to the paintings they felt were most iconic. These varied Australian works included stark portraits, scenes of the desert outback, colorful interiors, and a painting of dancers in a competition with numbers pinned to their dress jackets. First I conducted a painting tour with several people living with Alzheimer's that the educators watched and critiqued; then they conducted tours with other groups and I watched.

They faced a dilemma. How much do they teach about the paintings, how much do they present what they see in the paintings that they want the viewers to see, and how much do they encourage the participants to express what they see and feel about the art? This is not an either/or question. The awareness slowly dawned on the group that a shift was necessary in this type of tour from primarily teaching and convincing to enabling the people and viewers to look and express themselves.

When this happened, marvelous perceptions emerged. Participants saw right into the paintings; they seemed to see what the painters had in mind. One painting, called *The Flapper,* features a seated dancer from the early 1900s. The painter presents a seemingly well-composed young woman facing the viewer. Through a question-and-answer discussion, participants reached consensus that the upper part of the woman was that of "a proper lady." Then they noticed the model's crossed legs and stockings showing. They immediately remarked with strong moral judgment that when they were growing up, proper ladies sat with their legs together; never crossed. After discussing the difficulty of buying stockings in the war years, they agreed that the woman in the picture must be an actress or some other type of showgirl. Why else would she cross her legs in this suggestive way? The viewers clearly saw that the painter was presenting two sides of this woman, the proper and the risqué.

Another was called *The Drover's Wife;* a woman standing far from a covered wagon seems to be going nowhere. The audience sensed the emotion in the painting and saw immediately how uncomfortable the woman was. According to the art history of this painting, the woman in the painting had just found her husband cheating on her with a stable hand, and was walking away—but she had no place to go. The audience members said that the woman in the painting wanted to be anywhere but where she was.

These insights abound in tours of museums. In our research and preparation for the programs developed at the Louvre, the Museum of Modern Art, and the National Gallery of Australia, and for museums that are part of the ARTZ/McCance museum program in Massachusetts, the following artworks and objects were identified as increasing participants' focus of attention, engagement, and self-confidence.

LOUVRE, PARIS

The Card Sharp (*Le tricheur à l'as de carreau*), Georges de la Tour,
    1633–1639
Charity (*La Charité*), Jacques Blanchard, 1633
Cardinal Richelieu, Philippe de Champaigne, 1639
Peasant family (*Famille de paysans dans un intérieur*),
    Le Nain brothers, 1640
Peasants' Meal (*Repas de paysans*), Le Nain brothers,
    1642

MUSEUM OF MODERN ART (MoMA), NEW YORK

Christina's World, Andrew Wyeth, 1948

Agrarian Leader Zapata, Diego Rivera, 1931

The Sleeping Gypsy, Henri Rousseau, 1897

La Goulue at the Moulin Rouge, Henri de Toulouse-Lautrec,
    1891–1892

Girl with Ball, Roy Lichtenstein, 1961

PEABODY ESSEX MUSEUM, SALEM, MASSACHUSETTS

Portrait of George Crowninshield, Jr., attributed to Samuel F. B.
    Morse, 1816

Queen Elizabeth I, large-scale model, Basset-Lowke Ltd., 1949

Miss H., Douglas Volk, 1880

FULLER CRAFT MUSEUM, BROCKTON, MASSACHUSETTS

Waves, Yuko Nishimura, 2008

Radio Man, Gina Kamentsky, 2006

HARVARD MUSEUM OF NATURAL HISTORY,
CAMBRIDGE, MASSACHUSETTS

Whale skeleton

Gorillas

Hippopotamus fossil

Glass flowers

DeCORDOVA MUSEUM & SCULPTURE PARK,

LINCOLN, MASSACHUSETTS

Sunflowers for Vincent, Mark di Suvero, 1978–1983

Listening Stone, Joseph Wheelwright, 1995

Requiem to the 20th Century, 1936 Chrysler Air Stream,
  Nam June Paik, 1997

The Musical Fence, Paul Matisse, 1980

MUSEUM OF NATIONAL HERITAGE,

LEXINGTON, MASSACHUSETTS

Raggedy Ann doll, 1939–1949

Baseball glove, Draper-Maynard Co., 1920–1925

The Landing of the Pilgrim Fathers in America, A.D. *1620,*
  Charles Lucy, 1868

Benjamin Franklin, Joseph Wright, 1782

George Washington, Rembrandt Peale, 1847

NATIONAL GALLERY OF AUSTRALIA, CANBERRA

The Flapper, Margarte Preston, 1925

The Drover's Wife, Russell Drysdale, 1945

Sunday Stroll, Robert Dickerson, 1960

Interior in Yellow, Grace Cossington Smith, 1962, 1964

ARTS FOR HEALTH

The tour programs at the Louvre, at the National Gallery of Australia in Canberra, in the five Boston museums, and elsewhere, demonstrate how when art becomes an integral part of everyday life the quality of life for everyone living with Alzheimer's improves. The tours also make evident how great a paradigm shift is necessary to gain acceptance for and to implement such programs in cultural institutions generally. Accommodations and training are necessary, but they are only a beginning. The greatest challenge is to develop an attitude among such institutions that serving this group of people is a fundamental societal responsibility and can be meaningful to everyone involved.

One organization that has embraced the new paradigm is Chelsea and Westminster Hospital in London's Chelsea district. Its vibrant Arts for Health program has firmly established this approach in a hospital setting. Each of several large atria spaces in the hospital has a massive modern sculpture in its middle that patient rooms look out onto; hallways are covered with exciting modern artworks, and the hospital regularly hosts classical music concerts for patients, staff, and visitors. One special program offers professional artists wall space to display their artwork for sale—just as in a professional gallery.

And just as in a professional gallery, the hospital takes a percentage of the price of items sold as a commission.

In Vancouver, British Columbia, public art galleries have had shows of work by people living with Alzheimer's, and in eastern Australia several nursing homes with mostly Alzheimer's patients have engaged cultural artist Marily Cintra to develop "creative spaces" where residents' natural creativity is celebrated. This movement is only beginning—but it is already taking off.

The Bretonneau hospital in northwest Paris provides studio space for free to artists from the adjacent Montmartre area. In exchange, each artist agrees to spend several hours a week with patients of the hospital engaging them in artistic experiences. The hospital also has a fully equipped theater that it offers for free to local troupes for rehearsals and performances—in exchange for at least one performance of each play at no charge to members of the hospital community.

DO IT YOURSELF

In building your relationship with your partner, you can attend available programs in art institutions near where you live, planning outings to a different museum each week. If there are no programs near you, take this book to the museum access department and ask them to establish a program for people living with memory problems.

The other thing you can do is set up a program just for yourself and those you know—perhaps members of a support group. Here's how:

Identify a museum that your mother, for example, used to like to attend or a new museum that has exhibits you think might interest her, such as a local historical society. Ask the museum by e-mail or by phone if there is a special day of the week or time of day during which the museum is quieter than usual. Go to the museum store on your own and buy two dozen postcards of artworks on display that you think your mother might enjoy. When you get home ask her to choose the ones she likes best and ask why. Take notes. Revisit the museum in advance, see where each of the paintings, sculptures, historical artifacts, and photographs is located, and plan a tour in a naturally occurring sequence. If you think your mother will get tired and need a wheelchair or a strategically placed folding chair, arrange this with the staff beforehand. When you are in front of each artwork with your mother, ask her again what she feels, likes, and dislikes about each one. Use your notes from the earlier conversations as prompts. Have a wonderful time on your museum tour!

5

THE DRAMATIC ARTS

music, poetry, theater, films, and the circus

As soon as we hear a song that we haven't heard since a particular time in our lives, the flood gates of memory open and we're immersed in memories . . . a key unlocking all the experiences associated with the memory for the song, its time and place. —DANIEL J. LEVITIN

⚭ DRAMATIC ARTS differ from the visual arts because they touch multiple senses and thus different types of memories. They surround with sound, with sights, and with proprioceptive—body—experiences. It is harder in dramatic arts situations—in a theater, listening to music, or at the circus—to look away and turn inward. The dramatic ambience itself carries memory messages, even beyond the particular content. The rhythm and the beat of music are as engaging as the particular song. Recently a colleague asked, if familiar songs turn on people living with Alzheimer's, why does her father like listening to reggae music so much, which he never heard before? Rhythm and beat contain their own messages.

As with painting and sculpture, which people can enjoy creating themselves as well as looking at, the dramatic arts have the same allure. Listen to music or create it. Attend the circus or put on a clown's face and clown around yourself. Watch a play or write and act in one. Each engagement brings with it special challenges and joys. Each draws on unique brain abilities. Each can be part of your relationship building.

THEATER

Drama grabs the attention of people living with Alzheimer's, both when they are part of a theater audience and when they are acting in plays. Drama conveys feelings and ideas more forcefully than any formal lecture presentation can. Because those living with Alzheimer's understand and feel the emotions drama conveys, this mode of expression is a powerful way for them to communicate emotions related to living with Alzheimer's—their experience, their fears, and how they cope.

The *To Whom I May Concern* playwriting process results in an ever-changing, emotionally moving drama about the Alzheimer's experience written and performed by people living in the early stages of Alzheimer's. The developer of this process and the play's "author,"—gerontologist, nurse, and creative play-wright Maureen Matthews—generated the concept for such a drama in her doctoral dissertation at New York University. In focus group interviews with people who have lived with Alzheimer's for several years, Maureen captures their words, thoughts, and expressions. She translates these into a drama that members of the focus group eventually perform. During the development of this playwriting experience, Maureen worked with actor/director/social worker Lauren Volkmer, who is also an Artists for Alzheimer's volunteer, to rehearse and stage the play.

In an April 2006 production, performed at the New York City Alzheimer's Association's Early Stage conference, each of the four performers read letters written to doctors, to associations, and to God by people living with Alzheimer's, crafted from their words for emotional impact. Maureen and Lauren then developed visually striking staging in which the actors sat at simple tables with a large "letter bag" at the front of the stage.

Among the letters in the first public New York performance was one to a doctor who had delivered the initial diagnosis to one of the performers. "Probable Alzheimer's" was the diagnosis given, with the instruction to "take all this medicine and we just have to see what happens with it. And then come back in six months." "Will I be able to find my way here in six months? Will I be able to talk in six months?" the letter writer asks the doctor. The letter sarcastically includes the phone number of the local Alzheimer's Association that the doctor did not even have available when he gave her the diagnosis.

Another letter, from a man who went to Florida with his wife after his diagnosis, makes an important point about continuing to live with Alzheimer's. After complaining about how unhelpful the information he received at the time was to him, he ends with the salutation: "They're serving drinks on the patio . . . now there's something I can count on! See you when we get back. Confused in Florida."

One particularly moving letter is from a nurse who was refused membership in her professional association. She suspects it is because one member had told others on the membership committee she had been diagnosed with Alzheimer's:

Dear Sarah,

I must tell you that I'm very upset by the decision your organization made regarding my participation. As a retired nurse I was looking forward to the stimulating discussions and opportunity for learning that your group offers. I'm sure there is much that I could have offered as well as received. When I received word today that I was no longer wanted, I was devastated. Of course you didn't use those words. You said that membership was limited and you had already taken in your quota of new members for the year. But I saw one of your members' reaction when I shared with her that I had been diagnosed with Alzheimer's disease. How naïve I was that she would not be prejudiced and that she would communicate this to the membership committee.

I hope you will educate yourselves about the impact of Alzheimer's disease, especially for those in the early stages. I am still very much a part of the world and I'm not contagious.

Regretfully,

Margaret

Before standing for applause, each actor makes a personal statement at the end of the play about how he or she feels. Bob, one of the actors in that performance, expresses eloquently that he is very much still alive and engaged in life.

I still get excited about politics. I am concerned about the war in Iraq and hurricane Katrina and what's happening in Washington and Staten Island. I do have an opinion about President Bush. I do worry about the future of our country and our world. I also worry about my future.

I wrote another drama to convey to an audience that they must not stigmatize and hide away people living with Alzheimer's. It's also called *I'm Still Here*. Originally performed live, the play on video serves as the central feature to stimulate public discussion in a series of cable TV events that mayors of small towns in Massachusetts have sponsored. Together with the Hearthstone

Alzheimer's Care Foundation, each mayor develops a series of public talks, discussions, health fairs, and performances to raise awareness and provide information about living with Alzheimer's in his or her small town. The play's dramatic effect serves as a kickoff event for this local awareness process.

I'm Still Here, the play, follows a family coping with Alzheimer's symptoms and the eventual diagnosis of the father. It presents the reactions of various family members and colleagues as they become aware of the person's illness: fear, denial, anger, self-protection, and eventually understanding, love, and support. The play ends with the following monologue presented by the father at an Alzheimer's association event at which he admits his disease and lets others know he is still very much there:

Although I am no longer working as an attorney trying cases, I have a new calling of which I am very proud—to let as many people as possible know that living with Alzheimer's first means "living" and only second having an illness. Those of us with an Alzheimer's diagnosis still have a lot to contribute to our families, to those who are concerned about Alzheimer's, and to our communities.

Above all, I want to tell you: Don't avoid us! Don't forget us! Don't abandon us! The stigma of this illness stands in the way of all of us being part of society with respect and dignity.

And to conclude, as I said at the beginning of this speech, after the last very troubling year, and with a great deal of help from many of my old and new friends, I can finally say: "My name is Jim. I am a husband. I am a father. And I am a person living with Alzheimer's."

An audience member at one performance of *To Whom I May Concern* expressed clearly the role such dramas play in the lives of people with Alzheimer's: "Thank you for saying what we are all trying to say," he started, and then continued, "I have Alzheimer's and I am very much still alive with feelings, thoughts, and the need to express myself and stay engaged in life." Drama gets this message across eloquently.

POETRY

Poetry is an art form that also turns on parts of the brain that mere words do not. Both the reading and writing of poetry cuts across the brain's dysfunctions, enabling people living with Alzheimer's to engage fully—it touches parts of the brain that song also activates. While all poetry has these effects, dramatic poetry reading merges even further into the realm of theater.

Gary Glazner's Santa Fe Alzheimer's Poetry Project is an early and powerful effort to embrace poetry as a means of communication between people. He conducts dramatic poetry readings in assisted-living and nursing homes settings, as well as in public venues. His first public poetry event in New York City took place in early 2006 at the Bowery Poetry Club, a popular venue, where poets in the evening share their work. A collaboration of the club, the Artists for Alzheimer's program, and the New York City Alzheimer's Association, this event was organized for an audience that included people living with Alzheimer's and their partners. Gary Glazner, Bob Holman (who owns and manages the club), and I (who have been acting since I was young) were the major performers, dramatically reading from a book of poems that Gary and his Santa Fe project have compiled as particularly engaging to this group.

Students in Bob Holman's poetry class at Columbia University, along with members of the audience, read poems from Gary's poetry compilation. Toward the end of each public event a group poem is constructed with the audience and then dramatically recited. Gary constructs the poem from audience responses to the question: "What is the most beautiful thing you ever saw?" Everyone participates and everyone has a good time—there is no Alzheimer's in the room when the poem is read.

Here is a "most beautiful" poem that one of the groups at the Bowery Poetry Club generated with joy and enthusiasm:

It's a lot of things

It's all those things

I don't think of things that way

I'm too close to beauty

I don't get enough of beauty

I can't count them

Sunsets and so many things, it overwhelms me

Money

I see beauty very frequently

Like a mother and father picking up a child

It's their own child and they know it

It doesn't make any difference whether the child is good, bad,
*   or indifferent*

And I was a teacher, so I know

And if you get that right, you got that from me

They're so perfect

A sleepy black kitten is beautiful

Sunlight is the most beautiful thing I ever saw

I taught chemical engineering

The most beautiful thing I ever saw was fire

Ruth's eyes are beautiful

Sarah, my newborn daughter, good, bad, or indifferent.

My wife Virginia

Money isn't beautiful until you grow up

The sunset

A big yawn

What! What! What is beautiful!

Reading is beautiful

In New York City or in Turkey? The Bosphorus. Nothing in
*   this country compares with the Bosphorus.*

I don't know everything from today or tomorrow.

The beach in Jamaica

The stars

My mom is a beautiful woman

A spider in a spiderweb

Hearing sounds

Cat bird is a sound

The most beautiful thing I ever saw is you!

Traditional poems that people living with Alzheimer's selected as part of the Santa Fe anthology have certain characteristics, like the artwork that tends to be understood at the Louvre
and other museums. These poems are relatively short, to the
point, and contain strong images.

These are the characteristics of poems that work:

- Strong images
- Bold images of nature
- Possibly well known from childhood

- Short stanzas
- Short altogether

Gary's book includes many poems he has found that grab the attention of participants in the programs he organizes. As an ARTZ artist in residence, Lauren Volkmer also selected and tested poems with residents living with Alzheimer's. Those that had the most impact because they reflected the characteristics mentioned above were:

- Sonnet 18, William Shakespeare, 1609
- "The Tyger," William Blake, 1794
- "Daffodils," William Wordsworth, 1804
- "How Do I Love Thee?" (Sonnet 43), Elizabeth Barrett Browning, 1845
- "The Arrow and the Song," Henry Wadsworth Longfellow, 1845
- "The Owl and the Pussycat," Edward Lear, 1871
- "I Hear America Singing," Walt Whitman, 1860
- "I'm Nobody!" Emily Dickinson, 1870
- "The New Colossus," Emma Lazarus, 1883
- "Wynken, Blynken, and Nod," Eugene Field, 1889
- "The Road Not Taken," Robert Frost, 1916
- "Stopping by Woods on a Snowy Evening," Robert Frost, 1922

- "Sea-Fever," John Masefield, 1902
- "The House with Nobody in It," Joyce Kilmer, 1914

William Blake's "The Tyger" includes vibrant verbal descriptions of visual images and expresses strong emotions. Read dramatically, it is an excellent poem for this group.

Tyger! Tyger! Burning bright
In the forests of the night,
What immortal hand or eye
Could frame thy fearful symmetry?
In what distant deeps or skies
Burnt the fire of thine eyes?
On what wings dare he aspire?
What the hand, dare seize the fire?
And what shoulder, and what art,
Could twist the sinews of thy heart?
And when thy heart began to beat,
What dread hand? and what dread feet?
What the hammer? What the chain?
In what furnace was thy brain?
What the anvil? What dread grasp
Dare its deadly terrors clasp?
When the stars threw down their spears,
And water'd heaven with their tears,

Did he smile his work to see?

Did he who made the Lamb make thee?

Tyger! Tyger! Burning bright

In the forests of the night,

What immortal hand or eye

Dare frame thy fearful symmetry?

DO-IT-YOURSELF POETRY

You can write poetry with an individual living with Alzheimer's or with a group. While in public or community settings a professional writer might end up with "better" poetry, you can successfully write shared poetry by bringing to the practice your natural sensitivity to language and to the person. Poetry writing enables the person living with Alzheimer's and their partner the opportunity to express insights and to creatively use words. Writing poetry together requires few resources, affirms the worth of the person, and establishes relationship.

Individual writing results in a more consistent piece of work and the expression of a more personal vision. Here's the approach that John Killick, who initiated this process, suggests: If the person is not a close relative or friend, you first need to get to know her and gain her confidence. The confidence to be gained is her confidence in you at the moment, that if she speaks you are going to truly listen.

The first inviolable rule for poetry writing: Keep quiet and listen intently. It is too easy to fill a silence with your own chatter. Instead, give the person time to gather thoughts and feelings, and give her all the time she needs to find the right words and to utter them. Do nothing to interrupt that process.

When your partner starts to talk freely, ask permission to write down or tape-record their words. Never transcribe what a person says without observing first the common courtesy of asking permission.

Avoid suggesting a subject or giving any sort of lead. Just hold a conversation and listen. You are there to record and affirm, not to direct. You endow those words and the person himself with significance by the very act of writing down his words. Reinforce the message that you are listening with nods, yesses, and sympathetic noises of assent.

Do not try to construct a poem at this early stage in the process. The person is speaking prose and that's what you are writing down; it may also remain prose. When the person seems to have had their say, or is too tired to continue, stop. Disengage slowly and with consideration. Tell the person that you will bring a typed version of what they have said the next time you see them.

When you are alone and after you have typed up the text, read it carefully to see if the writings have any of the characteristics of poetry: rhythmic features, including repetition, and vivid emotional phrases, especially metaphors. If you find these, then there is the likelihood that there is a poem embedded in the prose. Rhyme is the least likely characteristic you will probably find, except occasionally and by accident, so don't spend a lot of time looking for rhyme.

If you find poetic characteristics, you are ready to begin creating poetry. Start by stripping away those elements that seem irrelevant or unhelpful to the main tenor of what you believe the person was expressing. Bring your own sensibility into play. But—and this is the second golden rule—at no point add anything. Every word in the eventual poem must come from the person. Remember, you are enabling—not interfering.

Bring the poem back to the person, read it to them and give them a copy printed out with 24-point type. If you ended up with a wonderful prose piece of writing, do the same thing. Ask permission to share the poem with others—family members, friends of the person, or staff. If the poem you found in the person's words is truly outstanding, ask if it would be possible to share it with a wider audience, such as in readings, radio broadcasts, publication in magazines or book form. If the person agrees, get an agreement in writing either from the person or from his or her representative. In the agreement be sure to determine whether the person's first or last name can be attached or whether the text should be attributed anonymously.

Where a number of poems have come from the same

individual—a family member or a person living in a community-based residential setting—consider publishing a pamphlet and holding a formal reading to which family and others are invited. Poems can also be framed and hung on the wall in celebration of the person's creativity.

STORYTELLING

Instead of poems, partners can also create stories together as a way of developing relationship. As psychologist Dan Schacter points out in his exceptionally readable book *Searching for Memory,* most of our memory skills diminish over time compared with those of younger people, but one remains stronger: storytelling. Perhaps because we tell and retell stories of our lives we tend to recall them. Even when we are old, others like to listen to the stories we tell—no matter how tied they are to actual memories or how we embellish them. As we age, with or without Alzheimer's, we often adopt the role of storyteller with our children and grandchildren. Anne Basting, building on this natural storytelling ability of elders, has developed an approach to relating to those living with Alzheimer's called TimeSlips.

While she focuses on storytelling and has developed a structured group approach to storytelling, Anne's insightful process reflects the fundamentals of sharing the dramatic arts with those living with Alzheimer's: how to talk and communicate, how to

present ideas, how to evoke creativity, and how to build relationships. Instead of listening to conversation and creating poems as
John Killick does, or interviewing people to write a play of
"letters" as did Maureen Matthews and Lauren Volkmer, Anne
encourages and trains people to develop stories—usually in a
group. What all these art experiences have in common is that
they focus on the person's abilities, they are essentially ways for
two or more people to relate to each other, and they bring joy
and fulfillment—principles for the dramatic arts with people
living with Alzheimer's.

Anne's process begins with setting the stage: the storytelling
facilitator reads the poem the group created previously, if there
is one, and then passes around a unique and often surprising
photograph—a baby sitting in an old leather doctor's bag, an
Annie, Get Your Gun woman in a long dress aiming a rifle along
railroad tracks, or a mountain climber leaping—almost flying—
between boulders over a deep ravine. Using this type of fantastic slightly unreal photo instead of natural snapshots enables the
person to imagine a story without the risk of being "wrong"
about facts that a familiar snapshot might pose. Naming a person
from a historical photo entails less risk than trying to guess
someone's name in a photo you might be supposed to recognize.
You risk being wrong.

In a group, everyone can look at a photo and can feel free
contributing a sensical or nonsensical phrase to the story being

made up about the photo, especially if someone else goes first. One person telling a story about the baby in the doctor's bag called him "Mischief." Another person in the group named the jumping mountain climber "Nutsy Gutsy." When people are enjoying themselves, they are less confused, less agitated, they initiate more conversations on their own, and generally are more communicative to family and friends. Why?

Anne convincingly reasons that people as they age increasingly discard and lose the social roles in life that define who they are: teacher, parent, friend, breadwinner. This does not mean that they cannot take on new roles and engage in new relationships. With Maureen and Lauren they became raconteurs, with Gary and John Killick they are poets. At the Louvre they become museumgoers. With Anne Basting, they become storytellers. In these new roles they feel empowered and useful; they replace memory with creativity.

All the arts experiences described in this book are successful when they build on the fundamental principle that as access to memory wanes in Alzheimer's, creativity remains vibrant and alive. Partners who firmly grasp this key build lasting and loving relationships.

In Anne's process a facilitator meets with a group of storytellers and, drawing on the ideas and words that the fantastic photographs bring to their minds, enables them to create entertaining and interesting stories. The facilitator asks questions, honoring and dignifying every answer. The facilitator might ask: What name would you give this person? When do you think this takes place? Where might she have come from? How long do you think he has been doing this? And every answer is okay; even multiple answers. Who says a person comes from only one place or has only one thought? Who says the various thoughts and names have to be aligned? All of us think thoughts that jump about. As a result the stories created in this way are fanciful, imaginative, fun, and creative.

Storytellers who are hard of hearing may not hear questions clearly. Similarly some museumgoers have trouble following what a guide says. A partner aware of this difficulty can help by sitting next to the person and repeating what is being said for the person to hear. Similarly, if a person has something to say but does not speak loud, the partner can amplify what she says to the rest of the group and the facilitator. Doing this is important in any of the arts experiences described here. Often participants are reticent to speak because they cannot see or hear what's going on, not because they have nothing to say. Anne calls those who help the person hear what is going on and amplify what the person says "echoers." Every art experience for people living with Alzheimer's needs an echoer to help with communication, especially in group settings and in public.

In order to reinforce the role of storyteller, poet, or actor, every art event needs to end with a celebration. The story, poem, play, or song is read and everyone is congratulated and thanked. Applause would not be a bad idea, either. Celebrating achievement in this way, whether it be reading the poem aloud when finished, submitting the poem to a local newspaper, or even framing it for the wall, gives the person and his or her partner joy and fun—improving mood and building relationship.

Because this form of storytelling was created for groups, if a partner wants to create a story at home, she might invite a group of friends to join in. The person living with Alzheimer's becomes one member of the group—each with different cognitive skills. Just make sure that those invited to join in don't fall back on memories and facts, but rather employ their own fun and fanciful imaginations.

If two partners want to generate stories together, they can start by sharing a photograph between them, interpreting it in their own way, and sharing their impressions with each other. The partner still needs to write down the story—and write brief notes rather than full sentences, to avoid upsetting the flow of storytelling. The partner also has to ask questions in a different way. Instead of asking, "What name would you give to the person in the photograph?" the partner can suggest an answer and ask for another: "I would call this person Crazy-Wazy, what about you?" Or, "I think this person is on her way to a wedding. What do you think she might find when she gets there?" The partner becomes one of two storytellers rather than a group facilitator.

In general, all the arts events described in this book are based on a deep understanding of what it is like to live with Alzheimer's, a desire to build a relationship with that person, and an understanding of the basic rules of communication between partners. The following list, slightly modified from one of Anne's, can serve universally as the rules of engagement between partners as well as between professionals and educators and people attending museums or other events.

- Approach the person from the front.
- Approach the person in an adult, not a childlike, way.
- Make eye contact.
- Match the person's eye level—sitting or standing.
- Begin by introducing yourself.
- Be calm.
- Speak slowly and coherently.
- Ask one question at a time.
- Give one-step directions.
- Allow time after you have spoken for the message to be heard and processed.
- Wait patiently for the answer; don't interrupt because you think the person has not understood.
- Reinforce your message with a gesture.
- Watch for nonverbal expressions.
- Don't interrupt the person when he or she is speaking.

- Repeat what you don't understand.
- Match the person's emotional tone when repeating what he or she said.
- Follow the person's lead in topics; let the person decide the topic rather than imposing topics you think are relevant.
- If asking for clarification by repeating the person's phrase, keep doing it with slight differences until the person tells you that you understood correctly.
- Validate the feeling the person expresses.
- Use touch to confirm feelings, but only if the person is open to it.
- Slow down your gestures and contain them; don't be too expressive.
- Explain your actions if they seem not to be understood.
- Avoid slang (unless the person's culture is part of the slang).
- Use words that relate to the person's age and experience.
- Enjoy yourself.
- Smile.

If you use this wonderful list you will have success most of the time communicating with those living with Alzheimer's, whether you are leading a museum tour, discussing films, or generating poetry.

MEET ME AT THE MOVIES:
A WALK DOWN MOVIE MEMORY LANE

Taking on the role of poet or storyteller is one way to be creative, develop skills, access memories, and be part of life. Another such role is that of moviegoer; but not just to any movie. ARTZ has identified a set of mostly Hollywood movies, musicals, and television scenes that seem to grab the attention of an audience of people living with Alzheimer's, as well as partners. The movies, the scenes themselves, and some of the actors are etched in many people's memories—and watching the scenes brings back the memories of having seen the film, of moviegoing moments in their own lives, of relaxing in the movies, and of feeling good about life.

The scenes do one more thing: they touch the emotions active in the person's functioning amygdala. What are these films, and why do they work? The following list is the result of extensive testing with residents and clients at Hearthstone residences and at the East Side Lenox House Neighborhood House in New York City. While the scenes and movies may seem evident and obvious once chosen, as do the paintings discussed in the last chapter, the scenes and the paintings are obviously the right ones only after they have been identified through research. When you create your own movie program at home, remember to try out a lot of movies and select the ones with lasting effect.

THE SCENE	THE MOVIE/TV SHOW	ACTOR/ACTRESS
"Oh, What a Beautiful Morning"	*Oklahoma*	Gordon MacRae
"Somewhere Over the Rainbow"	*The Wizard of Oz*	Judy Garland as Dorothy
"If I Were a Rich Man"	*Fiddler on the Roof*	Chaim Topol as Tevye
"I Am Dracula"	*Dracula*	Bela Lugosi
"Let 'Em Roll! In the Chocolate Factory"	*I Love Lucy*	Lucille Ball and Vivian Vance
"Plumbing Problems"	*The Three Stooges*	The Three Stooges (Moe, Larry, Curly)
"Singin' in the Rain"	*Singin' in the Rain*	Gene Kelly and Debbie Reynolds
"Do-Re-Mi"	*The Sound of Music*	Julie Andrews
"We'll Always Have Paris"	*Casablanca*	Ingrid Bergman, Humphrey Bogart, and Claude Rains
"The Richest Man in Town"	*It's a Wonderful Life*	James Stewart

The lives of the stars in many of these movies have been chronicled in fan magazines for years. Among these are Judy Garland, Humphrey Bogart, Lucille Ball, Ingrid Bergman, Gene Kelly, and

Jimmy Stewart. The same is the case for the movies themselves. Who has not heard of *Casablanca* and *The Wizard of Oz*?

But the most important feature of all these excerpts is the emotions each evokes: joy, anxiety, fear, sadness, hope, humor, silliness, love, regret, and relief are the ones that come to mind readily, although anyone who knows these movies might add a few more emotions to the list. What is the effect of evoking emotions? The person feels present and enabled. Everyone can laugh and cry equally well. Partners make connections at a deep, personal, and familiar level. At one recent showing, I witnessed a couple start out nervous and wary of making a mistake. By the end of the last scene they were sitting back, relaxed, holding hands just as when they were younger. There was no Alzheimer's in their relationship at that moment.

When I show these clips to groups, I generally get a colleague to join me. One of us sets up or "unpacks" each clip, and the other asks questions after the clip to both evoke and generate memories. A typical unpacking/setup goes like this, and by the time all the cues are given, someone in the audience has guessed what the movie is:

"The next clip you're going to see is from one of the most tender and yet saddest films I know. A real love story. What might that be? [Wait for an answer.] I'll give you a hint—it takes place in North Africa in World War II. In fact, the story takes place in a city with a casbah. One of the most famous lines from this movie is: 'Play it, Sam.' The movie stars one of the most famous actors of all time, Humphrey Bogart, that's right, 'Bogey,' and one of the most beautiful, Ingrid Bergman. That's right, the movie is *Casablanca*. Roll 'em."

After the final scene of the movie, in which Bogey persuades Bergman's character to leave him, and then protects her flight by killing the soldier trying to stop the flight, the memory-generating part takes place.

"Isn't that the saddest scene you've ever seen? It's also very tender and loving, isn't it? Have you ever been in love like that? Have you ever had to leave a loved one behind? And what war was that? That's right, World War II. Many people were in the army or lived through the war? Were you in the army, or did you know someone who was?"

By the time some of these topics have been answered, it will be time to introduce the next scene with: "And Sean [or Lauren] what's the next scene about?" Film programs can be conducted in groups or alone. They are better in groups, like storytelling, but they can also be created and engaged in by partners at home.

Go to the local video store and rent three old movies you think your husband might enjoy. After dinner put one in the player, tell him what the movie is about, in order to prime his memory, then watch it together. If he gets engaged in the movie, watch it to the end. If not, take it out and don't rent it again. After a month of evenings like this you will have identified a dozen favorites. Buy these or make legal copies and start your home movie library. Make a list of each movie with the plot and stars listed next to each title. Keep adding new titles to the list when you get bored with the ones you have seen a few times. Whenever you want to watch a movie together, ask which movie he would like to "go to" that evening. Read titles, descriptions, and stars from the list, let him choose—you can suggest a choice if none strikes his fancy—and have a fun time. Popcorn might be appropriate.

DO-IT-YOURSELF MUSIC AND PERFORMANCE

Do you, a friend, or family member play a musical instrument, sing, dance, take photographs, or like to paint? Invite all these people to "perform" for or with your husband. How well they do any of these things is not important. Eight people volunteering once a month enables you to have two "performances" a week. As much as the setting will allow, set up each event like a regular theater, lecture hall, or dance venue, even if it only means moving some furniture. Have someone you know prepare a "playbill" with the name of the "performer" and a short description of what she is going to be doing. Prepare refreshments for the "intermission." Have fun! Make a big thing of the performance during the day as well as when "the performer" arrives and makes her entrance. Everyone can have a good time and the person living with Alzheimer's will remember the happy emotions each time. Do not be surprised if she remarks at the third visit, "I've seen this before." She is not complaining, rather she is showing off and noticing that her memory is working better than before.

You probably know what type of music she likes best— classical, jazz, opera, rock and roll, country and western, crooners, musicals, religious hymns, marching bands, music of a particular era, the Beatles, Barbra Streisand, or Frank Sinatra. If you don't know which or you think she enjoys more than one type, start your music library as with the film library. Rent or buy a bunch of CDs and try them out. See which she remembers. Does she sing along with any particular song? Keep the ones that engage her; give the others away. Make it a point to play the music, talk with her about the performers, remind her of the good times that might be associated with the music, and enjoy yourselves.

If she likes opera or musical performances, don't be afraid to buy tickets to a nearby live performance and go together. Just be ready to leave at intermission or even earlier if she seems to be on edge. But don't be surprised if she stays focused for the entire three-hour performance. That's what I have found happens. If you do decide to leave, don't make a big thing of it. Make it seem natural and your decision. Be sure to go to the bathroom with her just before the performance and during intermission. If she says she doesn't have to go, remind her that there won't be another chance for a while. Use the toilet yourself if you have to in order to show her that it's really important and in order not to need to leave her alone at another time. So as to make going out fun for both of you, you want to avoid any chance of embarrassment in public for both her and you.

GET OUT AND ABOUT TOWN

Each of the creative dramatic art experiences described here can be carried out in a group, individually between partners, at home, in an assisted-living residence, at a nursing home, or in a day program. Although you can always bring art and artists to the person living with Alzheimer's, there is something special about doing it in reverse. Getting out, getting in a taxi or a car, arriving at the museum, poetry club, or movie theater is a valuable experience in itself and adds to the person's sense of self and sense of being part of society—of not being a societal discard.

One particular art experience almost requires getting out—going to the circus. Circus artists need equipment and a place to perform. Acrobats need trampolines and swings, jugglers need bowling pins and rings and a place high enough to toss them, horses and dogs need place to perform, and clowns need to be able to fall down, spray water on each other, and otherwise make fools of themselves. But, you might ask, isn't the circus too loud and too busy and too full of little children running around to be enjoyable to someone living with Alzheimer's?

The answer is no, it isn't? The Big Apple Circus in New York City has partnered with ARTZ, the Artists for Alzheimer's program, by donating groups of tickets annually and inviting people living with Alzheimer's and their partners from all over the city. The circus also makes sure that guides are available to help these special circusgoers get in front of the line, and that there are no stairs for them to climb. Everyone just loves it. They laugh at the clowns, are awed at the acrobats flying through the air, and sing along with the music. And they do this in the midst of shouting children, blaring noise, and more commotion than they have experienced for years—all without losing their attention for both halves of the show. When we went to see the Cirque Phénix in Paris with residents of the Bretonneau hospital, participants did the same thing—and the first half lasted an hour and a half. The high point was when one of the clowns belted out the "Marseillaise"—the French national anthem—on a trombone and one resident started conducting.

Why does circus art have the same effect as other art experiences, even under such seemingly harsh conditions? The circus—its sounds and sights and the way it feels—are familiar to all of us. The artists use their bodies to show off their skills and to tell stories. The noisy audience expresses its feelings with every "Ahhh!" and with every shout of glee or anticipation. All this viscerally makes sense to people living with Alzheimer's—in their bodies and minds. They don't have to think about it; they just know it makes sense—as the circus makes sense to everyone else.

The people in the circus also use facial expressions—especially the clowns. And we know that facial expressions of all kinds— joy, sadness, fear, and disgust—all register with people living with Alzheimer's because these expressions are hardwired in our brains. In fact, the entire experience, from entering the circus tent, to enjoying the spectacle, to leaving and reentering the quieter world, is familiar.

Above all, the circus is fun. We can describe the fact that the dramatic arts build on the procedural memory everyone is able to employ in learning throughout their lives, even with Alzheimer's. We can describe the way employing the creative part of ourselves makes us feel valued and empowered. We can speak of the social roles that attending and participating in art provides us with and how those roles are so important to our definition of who we are. All of that pales in comparison with the joy art brings to those with Alzheimer's and the sense of self they develop knowing that they are out and about in the city and taking part in the life they deserve. These experiences enable people to say "I'm still here" and to build relationships with one another because they are all part of the human condition.

6

TREATMENT BY DESIGN

how appropriate
living spaces encourage
independence and
well-being

The wall runs east to west; the peach tree grows flat against its southern side. The sun shines on the tree and as it warms the bricks behind the tree, the warm bricks themselves warm the peaches on the tree.

—CHRISTOPHER ALEXANDER

◯ WHEN I was studying for my doctorate in sociology at Columbia University, my mentor Robert Merton offered me a unique and special way to see the world. I instinctively knew that the set of "glasses" I was beginning to wear, as Merton called the viewpoint he shared with us, could also help create a better world. I found an immediate application for social science in designing environments to meet the needs of people in all sorts of buildings—housing suited to the cultural needs of immigrant groups, schools that accommodate children's play without becoming damaged and vandalized, hospitals that support healing as well as medical care, and offices that promote both health and efficient work. As the first Loeb Fellow in Environmental Design at Harvard's Graduate School of Design, where I remained on the faculty for nearly a decade, I had the exceptional opportunity to explore in depth the relationship among sociology, architecture, interiors, landscape, and planning.

This knowledge and experience fell into place many years later, when I was asked to find a new way to treat people living with Alzheimer's. I realized that if I could discover how physical environments help people in this extremely vulnerable group find their way and access their memories, these same principles could be used to create healthy environments of all sorts.

In fact, the designed physical environment can reduce Alzheimer's symptoms. In a multiyear study for the National Institute on Aging (NIA) we found that characteristics of the physical environment correlated with reductions in symptoms.

There are eight major characteristics of places that support people living with Alzheimer's to be all they can be: exit control, walking paths, privacy, shared spaces, gardens, homelike quality, sensory understanding, and supports for independence and empowerment. Below I discuss the design qualities to look for in residential settings that present themselves as Alzheimer's-competent. You can, however, take the same information and use it to look at your own home or the home in which the person lives with Alzheimer's.

EXIT CONTROL

Look for homes, assisted-living residences, and gardens that are safe and completely secure with unobtrusively locking doors, windows, fences, and other potential exits. Research has shown reduced depression among people living with Alzheimer's in settings with camouflaged exits that lead to places that may be dangerous. The hormone oxytocin is released in the brain when people feel safe. This in turn contributes to lower stress and to greater trust and sociability in such settings. In environments with secure and camouflaged exterior exits, partners and care staff can be more relaxed and can spend more time with residents.

WALKING PATHS

Look for destinations at the end of corridors and hallways that encourage walking rather than wandering. When the destination is clearly understood and visible, like a dining room or kitchen, the person knows where they are going. Landmarks located at points where a decision must be made, such as at a corner or going through a doorway, reduce the chance that someone with impaired way-finding will get lost. Elements that evoke what we believe to be hardwired memories and functions, such as music, smells of food, and a hearth are excellent landmarks. People with Alzheimer's walking on a path with a destination clearly are walking with more decision and direction than when there is no destination visible. Simple observation lets you know that. Our research, however, did not find that having well-planned walking paths was correlated with reduced agitation, aggression, or other symptoms we studied. We don't know why not. Further research is obviously needed.

PRIVACY

Look for private places with surfaces on which mementos and other personal objects that belong to the person can be easily displayed. Like everyone else, people living with Alzheimer's are more at ease when they have memory-evoking personal objects around them. There is a natural tendency for all living creatures to want some territory that is their own. Research clearly shows reduced anxiety and aggression as well as fewer psychotic symptoms in settings with greater opportunities for privacy and personalization. The safety, familiarity, and predictability of personal territory can also be linked to the positive effects of the body's calming oxytocin production.

SHARED SPACES

Look for kitchens, dining rooms, living rooms, and other group-activity spaces that look and feel different from one another.

Decoration and furnishings that clearly differentiate one place from another help promote appropriate behaviors in each room. When the environment tells us what is expected of us, we tend to hear it. Research shows that in settings where each shared space is decorated to evoke a different mood, people living with Alzheimer's are less likely to withdraw and isolate themselves. The desire to be with others, and to help and care for them, is a universal instinctive feeling that knowledgeable, creative design can evoke.

GARDENS

Look for porches, patios, and gardens that provide people living with Alzheimer's continuous and safe access to the out-of-doors. Such outdoor places ameliorate time-related disorders. Early in the progress of Alzheimer's disease people's internal sense of time is disturbed, resulting in sleep-wake disturbances, sun-downing, and other time disorientations. Physical contact with nature, and thus with the time of day, the weather, and the passing of the seasons helps people living with Alzheimer's remain aware of time passing. My own observations—as well as those of others—clearly indicate that gardens have positive effects, though it is difficult to capture these effects in research. Research is needed to determine the behavioral impacts of gardens taking into account physical accessibility, the presence or absence of horticultural therapy programs, the timing of doors to the garden being open or locked, and how safe the garden fence is. When you visit what is presented as an Alzheimer's-competent garden, look for these things as well. Just having a garden may not be enough to influence symptoms.

A HOMELIKE LIVING SPACE

Look for homelike environments. People living with Alzheimer's at home are already in a residential setting. Residential quality in assisted-living and similar group residences for people living with Alzheimer's can reduce symptoms. By this I mean homelike rooms that are not too big, with regular shape and familiar decor on the walls. There is little doubt that the territorial imperative, also linked to oxytocin, is centered at "home" for all living creatures. It is not surprising, therefore, to find that research shows reductions in both verbal and physical agitation in such settings.

THE FIVE SENSES

Look for environments that are designed so that people living with Alzheimer's glean the same information about the environment from what they see, hear, touch, and smell. Such settings are understood best. All living creatures employ all their senses simultaneously to understand their surroundings. If a kitchen is intended to be the social hub of a group, the more it looks, feels, sounds, and smells like a social hub the more it will be used that way. If a garden is to be used frequently, it needs to be inviting, highly visible through a window, and accessible through an easily located and unlocked door. The more fragrant, flowering plants there are, the more it feels like a garden. Each of us naturally develops coping strategies that triangulate our sensory awareness to compensate for diminished sight, hearing, or other sensory loss as we age. This is also true for people living with Alzheimer's disease. Research shows that where people have multiple sensory cues to understand the environment in which they live, verbal agitation and psychotic symptoms are reduced.

INDEPENDENCE AND EMPOWERMENT

Look for settings that are designed to enable people living with Alzheimer's to do by and for themselves things that foster independence, as much as possible. For example, walking is much easier when simple, inconspicuous rails to lean on are incorporated into a setting for support. The more the lean rail looks like a wide residential chair rail instead of an institutional grab bar, the better.

Bathroom doors that are highly visible with a readable sign, with toilet seats high enough for even those with weak legs to sit down and get up easily, ensure more frequent independent use. Safe, secure gardens with doors that enable views outside also invite independent use. Our minds naturally provide us with awareness of how our bodies relate to the environment, a process called proprioception, and maintaining a sense of control over our environment leads to a greater sense of empowerment.

In sum, wherever you and your partner live, if you find these eight characteristics, you will find a designed physical environment that profoundly influences how people living with Alzheimer's feel, behave, and function.

THE BRAIN AND THE DESIGNED ENVIRONMENT

These eight design characteristics were developed over two decades in the work of several researchers devoted to understanding how the needs of people living with Alzheimer's can be best met in design—M. Powell Lawton, Maggie Calkins, Uriel Cohen, and Gerald Weisman. My own approach to understanding why such design elements have the effects they do is to link them to cognitive mapping, way-finding, and memory—three brain attributes with which the neurosciences are concerned—and to two broader concepts, natural mapping and memory joggers.

Cognitive mapping is the mental process our brains employ

that enables us to remember paths connecting places we travel between. The more we find out about this cognitive activity, the more we realize that the fundamental factor in making cognitive mapping easy is the existence of landmarks by which we can guide ourselves. Because the brain's ability to develop a short-term cognitive map tends to be increasingly impaired over the course of Alzheimer's, the more an environment can provide hardwired cues to knowing where a person is, the longer he or she will be able to function there independently.

Way-finding is the mental and physical act of navigating through an environment—finding our way at night from our bed to the bathroom, finding our way from home to the store, or through an entirely new setting on vacation. Way-finding for most people is an unconscious process that uses procedural memory learning as a critical part of the process. In other words, if we take the same route over and over, it becomes second nature to us. The same is true for those with Alzheimer's, so the more clear and dominant a path is and the more multisensory cues indicate the pathway, the easier way-finding will be.

Memory is increasingly being studied by cognitive neuroscientists and psychologists. Memories are not like objects we store in a kitchen cabinet. They do not exist fully formed in a part of the brain into which we have placed them for later retrieval. Rather, attributes of experience are placed in different parts of the brain—faces in one part, colors in another, emotions related to an experience in another. Memories are retrieved, not by locating an entire experience in a cabinet in the mind and bringing it into consciousness, but rather by reconstituting the experience from the many places in which elements have been stored. Retrieval is like shouting to Scotty in *Star Trek,* "Beam me up, Scotty," and then having memories appear as do Captain Kirk and his crew, miraculously reassembled as whole persons.

Naturally mapped environments are obvious. A person in such a setting needs no map to find his way. Donald A. Norman developed this concept to identify why certain objects are easy to use, such as car seat adjusters in the shape of a car seat, and others difficult to learn, such as DVD players whose "time and date" function are notoriously impossible to figure out. For people living with Alzheimer's, the easier it is to comprehend and use an environment, the more empowered and independent they are there. Naturally mapped residential settings and gardens, with visible landmarks indicating destinations and turning points, give them the opportunity to find their way. While wandering is often seen as a "symptom" of Alzheimer's, it is more realistically a natural tendency that everyone has to explore, to search, and to have a goal. In a setting that has no obvious layout, people living with Alzheimer's *wander.* In a naturally mapped environment the same people *walk.*

Memory-jogging physical environments "cue" the person living with Alzheimer's to access memories embedded in his brain but that he may not otherwise be able to retrieve. Cues can be familiar photos on the wall such as pictures of seascapes and urban streets that remind people of the places they have spent their lives, "memory boxes" with life's mementos and achievements, and photos of children and grandchildren.

Memory cues can also be the person's own furniture in their original home, or in a group residential setting such as a special assisted-living residence for people living with Alzheimer's.

Both natural mapping and memory jogging elements let residents know what are appropriate behaviors in social and common rooms. In a living room, dining room, or kitchen, the silent language of decor makes evident the socially appropriate behaviors expected there—the room's natural mapping. The decor also jogs memories in that it reminds people of appropriate behaviors they hold in their brains—such as asking for tea and coffee in the kitchen, chatting with others in the living room, and sitting down to a meal in the dining room.

Alzheimer's is treatable, and the best treatment is one that carefully balances nonpharmacological with pharmacological approaches. Nonpharmacological treatment includes carefully planning and managing both the social and physical environment.

How do neuroscience principles apply to designing actual treatment settings in which people living with Alzheimer's and their families and friends feel comfortable? The following case study describes the application of these principles in an assisted-living treatment residence, which can be equally well applied to a family home.

The residence, located in the renovated Choate hospital in Woburn, Massachusetts, about twenty minutes north of Boston, houses twenty-six people with a twenty-four-hour staff. Twenty-four-hour staff means that there is always someone awake and willing to help with even the smallest thing, day or night. Some people spend only the day in the program, going home in the evening. Others live there. The residence is all on one floor and is secured with magnetic door locks that are deactivated either by coded push pads that allow only people who can remember the code to open the door or by a fire alarm in case of emergency. Entry doors that lead outside and doors used only in emergencies have no windows with views to the outside that might tempt residents to leave, and are the same color as adjacent walls. The door to the garden and the adjacent walls have many inviting windows to entice residents into this safe place. Surrounding the garden is a tall decorative fence providing complete safety. The fence boards jut up against one another, blocking out all views, to reduce agitation from activities beyond that might attract residents' interest and eventually lead to frustration.

A single straight corridor inside connects one end of the residence to the other so that no matter where residents are heading there is a destination visible. Frequent wall hangings provide an interesting and orienting walking path, including photographs of animals, children, seascapes, old cars, and flowers that residents have selected themselves and thus evidently understand; memory boxes with mementos of their lives; and decorated boards with announcements of events, staff members' names, and resident snapshots. At one end of the interior walking path is a fireplace/hearth and a living room with a television set where resident meetings are held and small group activities are organized. Almost at the other end is a common room with an easy-to-clean tile floor where residents engage in painting and other activities, and in the middle, one passes a large dining room and residential kitchen—separated by a half-wall so people can see in as they pass by.

Each common room is decorated differently to stimulate a unique mood in residents' minds. The living room, with white flowing curtains, is carpeted and has a decorative border near the ceiling. The kitchen/dining room has windows along one side, dining chairs and tables, a tile floor, and a residential kitchen with wooden cabinets and a breakfast counter. The faux-wood-floor common room adjacent to the porch and garden has less light, and furniture that can be moved easily to accommodate different uses. While not all residents may remember the precise attributes of each room, a functioning amygdala enables them to remember the "feel" of each and therefore to gradually develop patterns of use appropriate to each room.

Bedrooms provide residents the opportunity for privacy and personalization surrounded by their own furniture and mementos. All but six bedrooms have a bathroom just for the resident, while three two-bedroom apartments each have a bathroom used by the two residents. Everyone has their own furniture, wall hangings, and other decorations—all cues to improve memory and reduce agitation.

A wide outdoor porch adjacent to the common room provides a view over and access to a large garden. The covered porch is wide enough for chairs. Although it is cold in winter in New England, residents can still sit outside and look at the garden. A gentle ramp leads from the porch down to the completely enclosed and safe garden a half level below—carefully designed and landscaped with residential features and evidence-based way-finding principles established by planner-researcher Kevin Lynch. There is a clear walking path in the garden, along with planting boxes, benches, and landmarks to help residents orient themselves.

Each common room as well as each bedroom is scaled to feel residential. The ceilings are low, the furniture residential in style, and unique decorative borders on the walls near the ceiling reflect the use of each room. Everyone who lives, works, and visits there gets to know each other—to form a community. And because the residence has that many people, it has a real community feeling. In total twenty six residents, twenty-six staff over a twenty-four-hour period, and on weekends fifty family members and a dozen outside professionals such as doctors constitute a lively community of more than one hundred people. Some experts recommend residences of only seven to ten people each, but this can lead to boredom and staff stress and burnout, with only one or two people trying to keep a residence active and alive all day. Since boredom can lead to agitation and even aggression, I believe that a minimum size of approximately twenty-five residents is preferable for any treatment setting.

With finishes and fixtures that make the residence safe inside and with safety outside by virtue of secure doors and fences, residents are as independent as their physical capacity allows. Staff members, knowing that no one will get hurt or wander away, can relax and interact positively with residents because they do not feel they have to constantly prevent residents from doing what they want to do. There is an atmosphere of mutual support. A lean rail along hallway walls enables residents who might otherwise be unsteady on their feet to make their way to where they are going by themselves.

The residence is planned so that there are no strange sounds, views, or other confusing sensory stimuli. Furniture is familiar; the arbor in the garden is the same as in many residential yards;

the photos on the walls present comforting and familiar sights. There is no overhead public announcement system to confuse residents with random messages, and no strange and shiny floors waxed to meet regulations for cleanliness, as might be found in a long-term-care institution. The radio and television are not left on all day—programs are chosen and DVDs and audiotapes played that present familiar shows and tunes.

If you carefully plan or choose the physical setting in which someone with Alzheimer's lives, and take into account all these principles, your life and theirs will be easier. He or she will feel at home and as much in control as his or her age and physical condition allow. She will feel competent, and empowered, and exhibit fewer of the four Alzheimer's A's: less agitation, less anxiety, less aggression, and less apathy. The design and layout of residences for people living with Alzheimer's—their architecture, interiors, and landscape—can augment residents' memories and their ability to function independently. By accessing the parts of people's brains that are working well, and relieving stress on those parts that the illness affects, these settings support the whole person living there.

7

BUILDING A NEW RELATIONSHIP

the five rules of
communication and
the seven rules of
relationship building

Brenda, for her part, was able to hold on to Duncan; she remained in a living relationship with him, and it was in the safety of that relationship that she died. —TOM KITWOOD

NO MATTER how old and how healthy or ill, everyone needs social engagement and support to be as healthy as they can be. Rowe and Kahn's detailed MacArthur Foundation study of "Successful Aging" found that the healthiest people in old age have lots of friends, keep close contact with family members, participate frequently in social activities, and maintain other social links in their lives. Social relationships and supports are also necessary for those living with Alzheimer's who want a life with quality.

Social relationships can be seen as a treatment that reduces

Alzheimer's symptoms. A doctor or social worker writing a "social relationship prescription" would advise a person's partner to employ particularly emotive words and expressive body language, identify things to do that build on the person's hardwired memories, and create a schedule that fills the person's day with meaningful activities. While doing this might take up all of a partner's day, even moderately filling such a prescription will yield immense benefits.

Communication starts with mutual understanding. Every partner in relationship with a person living with Alzheimer's—spouse, paid caregiver, friend, medical professional, social worker, or family member—needs to understand the meaning of their own and the other person's communication within the context of what is known about the brain during its progress through Alzheimer's. In the beginning, there may be some difficulty with words and concepts. Later on, the person may seem illogical. To develop and maintain a relationship in Alzheimer's, partners need to keep in mind that whatever is said, the person living with Alzheimer's does not hear herself "making no sense." Whatever others hear, the person internally hears sense.

My colleague and friend Paul Robertson, founder and former first violinist with the world-renowned Medici quartet, taught me a musical expression for this state of mind. In a performance program we developed, called Swansongs, he demonstrates internal sense and the lack of external understanding by

first playing very sweetly a well-known Mozart composition—
"Twinkle, Twinkle, Little Star." Everyone in the audience knows
the tune and feels comfortable with its structure and closure.
Then Paul changes one string, in a technique known as scor-
datura (Italian for "mistuning"), on his remarkable 1726 Mon-
tagnana Venetian violin, and plays "Twinkle, Twinkle, Little
Star" again. Except this time, the exact same bowing results in a
different and, to the listener, "distorted" tune. While the listener
recognizes the original melody among the discordant set of
notes, she also recognizes that there is something wrong. The
person living with Alzheimer's is the violin. She knows she is
playing "Twinkle, Twinkle, Little Star" and may or may not
hear the discordant notes. The listener has a choice; either to
correct the violinist—the person living with Alzheimer's—
pointing out how badly she is playing, or to hear the music that
is intended and respond appropriately.

There is a term for such responses: phatic communication.
Phatic sentences, utterances, and sounds are used in daily conversation to express friendship, social responsiveness, and caring,
rather than to convey information. How many of us are really interested in the details of another person's state of mind when we
ask, "How are you?" And do we really want a response from the
other person when we shout: "Hey there!" We tend to converse
about the weather, sports, and old friends, to make social contact
with others. Phatic communication recognizes the other person's

presence, and makes a connection, without requiring a lengthy response. Coined by the anthropologist Bronislaw Malinowski in the early 1900s, the term has the same root as "aphasia," the loss of the ability to understand language, a problem some people with Alzheimer's face. Phatic conversation is an excellent way to communicate with people living with Alzheimer's who remain in touch with what they feel, who appreciate staying in touch with others, and who even understand what they mean to say—even if the words are difficult to come by.

THE FIVE RULES OF COMMUNICATION

Hear and respond to the other person's "reality." Early in the illness there may not be a great difference between the realities of the two partners in the relationship—just greater difficulty on the part of the person with Alzheimer's to put all the pieces of "reality" together as quickly and as surely as before. A person may know it is the weekend, but not have a strong memory of how the previous week has passed or what the following week will be like—something another person might use to frame his picture of "weekend."

Later on in the progress of Alzheimer's, different definitions of "reality" are more pronounced. Nevertheless, people who live with Alzheimer's may not know that the person they are talking to has a different definition of reality than they do. Waking in the middle of the night thinking it is morning, a person acts on his reality that it is morning without being aware that someone else might think it is midnight. If he believes a relative who passed away years before is arriving to accompany him on a trip, that is his reality. If he feels that other people are treating him badly or that he has had nothing to eat recently, that is his reality.

When others attempt to get someone to change how they see the world—whether the person is living with Alzheimer's or not—the reaction is predictable: anger, resistance, and withdrawal. It would be as if someone persistently tried to convince you that you are actually a citizen of the moon, and refused to stop no matter how much you objected. At some point your patience would wear thin and you would reply in anger, "Leave me alone!" It is kinder and much more respectful to understand and respond to whatever reality the other expresses. It also reduces anxiety and aggression and is therefore a successful form of treatment.

This is not dissimilar to our own daily lives. When is the last time you responded to an upset friend who was complaining, "I am having the worst day of my life," by saying in return, "No, not really. The worst day was probably two years ago when your father died in a car crash"? You wouldn't think of saying anything like that because you know it would only upset your friend more. The other person would only get more angry, anxious, and unhappy—all directed at you. This is the same effect that correcting the reality of a person living with Alzheimer's has on her. At that moment for both your friend and the person living with Alzheimer's, it is the worst day of their lives.

Partners who can respond to the feelings underlying what another is saying can reduce anxiety, agitation, and aggression.

Be honest. While we are all aware of other people's feelings, people living with Alzheimer's disease are exquisitely sensitive to the feelings of others—including whether they are being honest or dishonest. Some people interpret honesty to mean expressing every attitude and feeling they have, even telling the other person that they are wrong when the person says something that is clearly false—for example getting the day of the week wrong. Correcting the person each time you see things differently is no more honest than responding to that person's reality. Honesty means being yourself. The person living with Alzheimer's is likely to be more at ease—less anxious, agitated, and aggressive— when the person with whom he is in relationship is straightforward and being herself. From this point of honesty a person can correct the one who thinks night is day by expressing her own reality, "I believe it's the middle of the night." This way of presenting your truth is nonconfrontational and respectful. Others have their truth; you, yours.

Another form of honesty, emotional honesty, is also a part of a healthy relationship between a person living with Alzheimer's and others. If someone is sad or happy and expresses his feelings, the person living with Alzheimer's will respond appropriately. A person living with Alzheimer's whose amygdala is working well—as most people's are—feels particularly good when he can express a feeling, whether of concern, empathy, fear, or love. When you honestly express your feelings, he can do this honestly as well.

Honesty includes responding with empathy to the person's definition of reality. It is not a lie to feel concern when a person cries about being abandoned, even when you know in fact she is being cared for compassionately. She feels abandoned—perhaps because she can't remember that you have been with her recently, or because she knows deep down that the disease is making her more dependent. It is not dishonest to deal directly with that feeling of abandonment. Some people call going along with the person's definition of a situation without correcting the reality a "fiblet—a little lie." Not telling someone that the husband she is waiting for died years ago is no more a lie than not correcting your spouse when she says it was the worst day of her life.

Always address the person directly. No one likes hearing people talking about them as if they were not there. In every situation be sure to talk directly to the person living with Alzheimer's. This point is made with humor and pathos in a wonderful play and movie, D. L. Coburn's *The Gin Game.* In one scene, two older people (played by Hume Cronyn and his wife, Jessica Tandy, in the moving original 1977 production) are playing cards—gin rummy, of course—and talking about why they hate being in a nursing home.

> *HE:* "I hate it when people say, 'Are we hungry for dinner now?' when they mean 'Are you hungry?'"
> *SHE:* "I feel even worse when they talk about me in the third person to someone else, and I'm sitting right there: 'Do you think she needs a bath?' they ask another nurse."

The person is there. The person knows she's there. It is up to others to remember and recognize this always. As the disease progresses, other people increasingly are the keepers of that person's personhood. Those who overlook this contribute directly to the person's anxiety, agitation, aggression, and apathy. Acknowledging the person by words and actions reduces these symptoms.

Even professionals can get it wrong. In a Public Broadcasting Service television special called *The Forgetting,* one scene takes place in a doctor's office. The doctor is giving advice to an older couple in which the wife is living with Alzheimer's. Throughout the scene the doctor addresses all his remarks to the husband, ignoring the wife's presence—as if she could not hear what was being said, as if she could not understand, as if she were not there. "Does your wife get up at night?" "Have your wife take these pills." The impact of being treated as if she does not exist is abundantly evident in the wife's body language—she sinks into apathetic passivity.

Don't test! Everyday we ask others for information and data—sometimes because we don't know the answer, sometimes because we want to check on a fact, and sometimes because we want to test the other's knowledge. "Do you remember the name of that famous actor in *Gone With the Wind*?" "Who was it we had dinner with last month?" "Look at this picture of our wedding. Can you tell who this is?" The term "Can you" is a test question that always needs to be avoided—Can you tell me? Can you remember? In normal situations, such questions may be okay—although as I get older and have greater difficulty remembering certain specifics, I wish others would ask me questions like this less often.

For a person living with Alzheimer's, from the very beginning of the illness, posing such questions feels increasingly like a test of memory they are sure to fail. The person living with Alzheimer's wishes he were the same person he always was. We all wish he had the same access to memory he always did, the same recollections, and the same skills. In search of these former skills, partners often test the person. "Remember me?" a son might ask. Pointing to a grandson, he asks, "You know this little fellow's name, don't you?" Every time a person is tested, he is made aware again that he is losing a grip on reality. He recognizes the child as a relative he loves, and knows that he ought to remember the child's name, but he can't. Every test is a reminder of failings and losses. Every test increases the person's feelings of inadequacy.

Why do we test? We test to make ourselves feel better. We want to know that we exist in the person's mind as we have always existed. We want the person to recognize and enjoy her grandchildren as she always has. While we say we are testing to help the person enjoy her world, testing puts each event into our context, not hers. Each "correct" answer relieves us of our apprehension and guilt that we are not doing enough for the person we love. Each "wrong" answer makes her feel bad about herself. We can do better. We can avoid testing for knowledge that the person doesn't have readily accessible. We can avoid testing for executive function skills that are lost.

If we are more interested in the relationship and the person's enjoyment, we can give him the answers rather than ask questions. This achieves the same results while decreasing anxiety and agitation. A son might introduce his own son to his grandmother by saying, "Hi, Mom, this is your grandson Adam who you always enjoy singing songs with." Such an introduction gives her all the information she needs to be socially appropriate, access relevant memories, and be the person she always has been with her grandson. Such an approach makes her feel competent and in control. This is a critical form of Alzheimer's treatment. Adam can also wear a name tag that says, "I'm your grandson Adam and I love you."

Don't say "don't"; divert and redirect instead. A person living with Alzheimer's doing something silly by mistake or something inappropriate or dangerous is not likely to realize what he is doing. If he wants to take a walk, he may not understand why that is dangerous. If he wants to cook a meal and turns on the stove, he probably does not think this is dangerous, because he doesn't think he may forget the pot and not turn off the stove. He doesn't realize the side effects of his actions—getting lost in an unfamiliar place or setting the house on fire. He therefore cannot understand when another person tells him not to do what he is doing. "Don't!" doesn't mean anything to a person who does not understand why he should not do something. And explaining the reason may not help. Telling someone who doesn't know he has way-finding difficulties that he might get lost in his own neighborhood falls on deaf ears.

Instead of saying, "Don't do that!" it is kinder and more effective to change the subject so that the person focuses on something else, and then to suggest another attractive and safer alternative. This is what it means to divert and redirect. Diverting the person's attention from an inappropriate action onto an-other subject (divert) and then attracting him to another, safer ac-tivity (redirect) tends to work best. If he wants to take a walk in an unfamiliar environment that might be unsafe for him, and if his partner can't at that moment join him for the walk, which is always preferred, the partner might divert him with a comment about the weather and then redirect him to a cup of tea or coffee.

Redirection feels like pressure to someone who is moving steadily ahead. If you are headed for the door at the end of a party and someone asks you not to leave so soon and actually stops you from going, you may get annoyed. But if you are stopped by someone asking about your kids' music lessons or by the sudden clatter of pots being dropped in the kitchen, and then asked about your children, there is less likelihood of being annoyed. That's why, with people living with Alzheimer's, it is essential to create a diversion first before suggesting a more ap-propriate or safer activity. When I discussed this principle with a group in a workshop at the annual North Shore Alzheimer's Partnership, near Boston, one participant gave me a memorable example. Her husband with Alzheimer's was watching tele-vision. They were both in their eighties and it was time to go to bed. No matter what she said, her husband wouldn't budge. So she went into the bathroom and came back into the living room stark naked—a diversion. It was then a lot easier to redirect her husband from the television to bed.

THE SEVEN RULES OF RELATIONSHIP BUILDING

Communication is the building block of relationships. Other building blocks include understanding and embracing the other person for who they are. It is automatic for some partners to correct the person living with Alzheimer's if he is behaving oddly. This section is not about changing the other person's behavior, it's about changing your own. It describes how you can modify the way you react so that you don't make matters worse by instigating the precise behaviors in the person that you want to avoid.

Don't be a rock—respond, don't react. Woody Widrick, minister of the Unitarian Church in Carlisle, Massachusetts, used to give a sermon once a year on not being a rock. If you kick a small rock, he would say, it reacts, it moves. It doesn't think; it just goes where you kick it. Whenever people react to situations without thinking, they are behaving like rocks. Being a rock in relationship with people living with Alzheimer's means that when they get angry, you get defensive and angry back. When they repeat themselves because they can't remember the answer to a question they just asked, you get frustrated and tell them to stop being so tiresome. When they say they're going for a walk and you know that they will get lost even though the walk is just in the neighborhood, you lock the door to keep them inside. When they drop their food, you admonish them for being like a child.

These extreme rocklike reactions happen more often than we realize. And when they do, the person living with Alzheimer's gets more anxious, more agitated, and runs the risk of becoming aggressive—three of the big four A's.

How can people train themselves to respond rather than react? They can start by inserting their own mind between the other person's actions and their own reactions. This means engaging their own hippocampus in lieu of the other person engaging his. Remember that the hippocampus together with the orbitofrontal cortex and thalamus prevents us from reacting to everything around us as if there were no secondary or tertiary consequences. We don't smash our car into every other car that cuts into our lane on the highway. We don't scream every time we hear about an atrocity committed in another country. In these cases, we autonomically engage our hippocampus, orbitofrontal cortex, and thalamus, which say to us, "Think a second. Do you really want to pay for the damage to your own car? Do you really believe that screaming will change the situation?" When we are small children, we react more than we respond—we are rocks. As we become adults, we respond more and more and react less and less. What people living with Alzheimer's need us to do in our relationship with them is to stop being rocks and behave like people.

Responding is treatment. When the person asks the same question over and over, one positive thing to do is answer over and over with no emotion, without getting impatient. Another even more positive thing to do is to give the person a note with the answer written clearly on it in large letters, and each time they ask the question to remind them to look at the note for the answer. When the person gets angry at you for some event you feel is imaginary, try to control yourself—whatever you do, don't get angry back. Don't escalate the anger. Even though you think you did nothing, apologizing and promising never to do it again will diffuse the tension. All these are thoughtful responses to difficult situations, rather than rocklike reactions. Each measured response contributes to reduced agitation and aggression. Each measured response is treatment.

Be present! This admonition is like a Zen Buddhist wake-up call. Pay attention! Remember yourself! Be aware! Wake up! What does this mean in relation to a person living with Alzheimer's? How can paying attention be treatment? The answer is simple. Because of an increase in emotional sensitivity of a person living with Alzheimer's throughout the illness, everything you do when in their presence affects them. When you smile or frown, when you pay attention to what is being said or have your attention diverted, when you talk about something important or unimportant—all these actions directly affect the relationship.

If you and a friend go out to get ice cream with the person

who has Alzheimer's, it is likely the person will react to the complexity of the physical and social setting, not to you. She will probably be thrown by the strange environment, difficult choices to make, two people talking about topics she understands little of, and lots of interesting activity on the street outside the shop window. She will look out the window, interrupt your conversation with seemingly incongruous observations, and otherwise be disruptive. In the ice cream shop you are not present to her, so she is not present to you.

On the other hand, if you move to a simpler place and focus your attention on her—she will focus back on you. Your behavior will affect hers; even the slightest nuance. When you are with a person living with Alzheimer's in this way they are totally with you. Their minds are not wandering to other subjects. As in a Zen frame of mind—there are no other subjects floating around in their minds. Farther into the illness, they may not even be thinking about the future, which may by then have less reality to them. They are not thinking about something else to do, because you are there and you are what they are doing. You are important.

Whatever you do or don't do in the immediate one-to-one relationship defines the situation for that person. If you remain present through the entire interaction, the person will too. If your mind wanders, so will the person's.

Being present to the situation also means that you are present to the person himself. Being sensitive to each expression and mindful of every nuance of his behavior improves the chance that you will be able to respond rather than react to what he does. Being present means that you are less likely to do something without thinking that upsets the person. You are less likely to startle him or ask questions he can't answer. In the same way that lovers are present to one another, being present to a person living with Alzheimer's expresses tenderness, caring, and love. The person, sensing these emotions, relaxes with less agitation, anxiety, and aggression. Treatment!

Do as little as possible to help the person be successful—but leave nothing undone. The more we do for someone, the less they do for themselves. The more we help our children with their homework, the more dependent on us they become and the less they learn. The more we do for our friends when they are in emotional trouble, the more dependent they grow on us and the less they learn how to get themselves out of such trouble the next time. Learned helplessness of this sort also occurs with people living with Alzheimer's.

When dressing, bathing, eating, grooming, walking, and so on, people living with Alzheimer's slowly but surely need more and more help. At every stage, the demand for help is greater. At the start, a reminder might suffice. Later on a set of written instructions might be needed. Eventually a helping hand is necessary. Often partners, wanting to do the right thing, say to the person they love, "Leave it to me. I'll do it for you." Don't say this! Fill in the blanks. Organize the steps and let the person carry them out. Do only what is needed. The more you do for the person, the faster they learn that helplessness is the best policy. The less they do, the more you do, and the easier it is for them to slip into apathy.

Inversely, the more a person is self-sufficient—the more pieces of a complex task she completes herself—the more successful she feels. Success breeds success in every activity of daily living as well as in more complex endeavors. The old dictum "use it or lose it" holds true for people living with Alzheimer's. In the flow of daily life, the more a person does for himself, the more successful he is. The more the person controls the outcomes of his actions, the longer these skills last in his life.

Use all the senses. Don't talk so much. As when someone has a hangover, too many words give him a headache. The person with Alzheimer's gets a headache from too many words, not because he drank too much the night before, but because his brain's Wernicke's and Broca's areas—the language centers—aren't working well. It is more difficult for him to pay attention to words. But, like everyone living with Alzheimer's, he can still use all his other senses to put together a relatively coherent picture of the state he is in. Whether or not the words "Dinner's ready" make sense, nonverbal sense-related cues can adequately convey that it's dinnertime: the smell of a chicken in the oven, the feel of steam in the room from boiling potatoes, the sound of dinner plates and cutlery as the table is being set, awareness of activity in the kitchen, being asked to change for dinner, and given a taste of soup to "test." Don't mask these odors and sounds, broadcast them.

A hug, a rub on the back, and a kiss always convey love and affection better than words do. If you want to take a walk with someone, put on your overcoat first and get hers out before suggesting a walk. Use sounds, sight, tastes, odors, hugs, touching hands and textures, and sensations of warmth and cold to communicate. Then if that doesn't work, use words.

Find the person's doodling. As we age with or without Alzheimer's disease we retain certain fine and gross motor skills that we associate with who we are—with what makes us unique. I doodle. When I have nothing to do with my hands or am listening to a lecture and have my mind engaged but not my fingers, I make abstract line drawings that express a mood or a situation.

I have been doodling for years and expect to be doing so for years to come, no matter how old I am. I have collected my doodles for years and have put them in a scrapbook. I will recognize and be intrigued by them when I am old.

Everyone has his own unique doodles. By "doodling," I mean a wide variety of self-expression. Doodling includes knitting, playing the piano, reading aloud to others, painting, and even working on a computer. Each person has his own specialty. Finding those unique skills and invoking them through shared activities engages that part of a person that relaxes him and enables him to soothe himself.

For eighty-four-year-old Mary Spencer of Gillette, Wyoming, it's bowling. When Mary bowls she doesn't have to think about how to hold the ball with three fingers, how to swing her arm back to gain momentum, or how to bowl strikes. She knows how. This complex sequence—from picking up the bowling ball to celebrating a strike as the pins drop—is second nature to her. Repeated years of practice have embedded the know-how Mary needs to bowl like the experienced bowler she is, in the procedural memory part of her brain and in her body. When Mary bowls, she is not confused, she fits in, and she enjoys herself; there is no Alzheimer's in the bowling alley. As the Gillette *News Record* reports:

> *Mary Spencer takes small and tentative steps toward the foul line. She holds an orange bowling ball in hands as finely boned as the cartilage of a bird's wing. Several feet from the foul line she lifts her head and sights down the lane at the arrangement of pins. She takes a small sidestep to the left and aligns herself.*
>
> *The ball begins a slow arc toward the gutter, leans precari-*

ously over that precipice of failure, then follows the arc to its conclusion—the center pin. Nine go down with wooden clatter and fanfare in the dim, smoky alleys of Camel Lanes.

"Whoo," a few of her teammates cry. . . .

Spencer turns a lot of heads when she bowls.

They may not know she's bowled for half a century. Or that her olive skin was inherited from her mother, a full-blooded Iroquois named Princess Clearwater. Or that she was a regular "Rosie the Riveter"—rolled-up shirtsleeves, brawny arms and all—during World War II, wiring cockpits for Lockheed while her husband served in the Army Armored Division.

The way she bowls, they probably wouldn't even guess she has stage two Alzheimer's disease. . . .

She returns from the lane with a strike in her belt and bowling a good game. Spencer gets up from the table and makes her way over to the bowling balls. She picks up a green hand towel from off the rack and rubs the ball down, just the part near the finger holes. It's a ritual she completes every time. . . .

Even at 84, she's out-bowling most of the women on the team. That stroke is so ingrained into her joints and tendons, and into her most primal memory, that even when all else begins to blur, the names and faces of those closest to her, her bowling is as sharp as ever.

THE PRINCIPLE OF "I" IN THE "WE"

The Buddha said to his disciples, "Our actions are our only possessions." Another way to say this is that everything we do is part of our definition of who we are. Because few people living with Alzheimer's have a job or some other socially prominent position by which to develop a strong self-image and thus define themselves, the more others do to help them achieve this, the greater is their sense of self.

Studying spiritual growth under many conditions teaches us that a significant part of our spiritual quest and personal growth is to understand who we are within a greater collective whole—the "I" in the "we"—and how these are connected.

This message came to me forcefully from my daughter Isabelle, who worked intermittently for several years as an activities program director in a Hearthstone assisted-living program for people living with Alzheimer's. One day she came home and exclaimed that the lack of a balloon had taught her a critical communications lesson. What happened? I asked her. Residents sometimes play a game that might be called Tap the Balloon, she said. Sitting in a circle they tap an inflated balloon to the center of the circle or to each other. Tap the Balloon requires both visual acuity and physical motor skills. But there was no balloon to be had anywhere that day. Instead, Isabelle picked up a large beach ball usually used in the garden. She saw changes greater than she had expected.

Rather than tapping the large ball, each person had to catch it. When they caught it, Isabelle congratulated them *by name* with a "Well done!" and suggested another person *by name* to whom they should pass the ball. Instead of the impersonal and nameless "tap," the new game included a personal "catch and throw" in which names were used. Isabelle remarked, "Everyone was more involved because they heard their own name and recognized the other people in the circle also by name. The game," she told me, "shifted from tapping a balloon into the air, to one in which each person purposefully tossed a ball to another who had a name too." By selecting an object that each person had to grasp and then throw purposefully to someone else, Isabelle had discovered a basic human principle of spirituality—one that helps immensely in Alzheimer's treatment.

Every social event can include these two elements. When people sit down to dinner, the one arranging dinner can address them by their name or reference ("Hi, Maisie" or "Hi, Mom") and introduce them to their neighbor at dinner ("How about sitting next to Karin this evening?" or "Do you want to sit next to your grandson Evan"). The principle of "I" in the "we" can permeate every relationship.

FOLLOW THE FLOW OF THE DAY

A person living with Alzheimer's who enjoys doing things may find it burdensome to plan a sequence of tasks to do to keep herself busy all day long. Providing the person a daily flow of things to do that engages her mind, body, and spirit helps her live a more normal life.

Characteristics of the flow of the day may be hardwired in the brain or learned from lifelong routines. Our brains have a higher level of the neurotransmitter acetylcholine in the morning when we wake up, so we have greater energy than when we go to sleep at the end of the day. Usually we are hungry three times a day—although this may be more cultural than hardwired. Meals are generally preceded by preparation and succeeded by cleaning up. Preplanning and "shopping" are part of longer-term meal preparation. In our daily lives we have social contact with others—family, friends, those with whom we have commercial interactions, and even strangers. Some of the things we do require us to engage actively, to participate, while we may engage in other activities passively—watching and enjoying. Some things we do for relaxation; others for exercise. Some things engage our aesthetic capacities; others engage us spiritually. The flow of the day has its more active and less active times. In the evening we get tired and go to sleep.

The more the day of a person with Alzheimer's naturally reflects the regularity of a usual day as well as its complexity, the more the day and its activities will engage him, keep his attention, and reduce anxiety, agitation, aggression, and apathy. In other words, the more natural the day, the more the day is treatment for the disease.

8

APPRECIATING THE NEW RELATIONSHIP

accepting the changes
in a loved one living
with alzheimer's

My memory of it could arise from the difficulty I now feel in writing about Iris as she was. Is it that I think of her only as she now is, which is for me the same as she has always been? —JOHN BAYLEY

◊ WHENEVER MAJOR CHANGE disrupts any relationship— disability, or moving from one stage of life to another— everyone involved has to build a new relationship with the other if the relationship is to continue and flourish. This is the case as well when a person begins to live with Alzheimer's. At that juncture, partners have a choice to build a new and dynamic relationship with the person living with Alzheimer's, or not. Many people make the latter choice.

In a healthy parent-child relationship, each time one person goes through a major life change, both have to develop a new relationship. I developed a new relationship with my children when each moved from being a dependent child to a teenager to an adult. In one sense, they remain my children; in another sense, they have become adults to whom I must relate as an adult. Sometimes this change in relationship was forced on me—each child insisted forcefully, more often in actions than in words, that I be different in our relationship. They had changed; I had to change too. Such a shift in relationship at each of life's passages is a transformation we all experience. Usually, the transition is a happy one. The child becomes an adult; I have a friend as well as a dependent. The child has children; I am a grandparent. My colleague was promoted; I have a friend in a new position of influence. My wife got her Ph.D.; I have a professional partner and we have to have a different set of work/family relationships because of the new opportunities that lie before her.

Sometimes these transitions are less joyous. A woman realizes that her son is addicted to heroin and has to express her love in a different way. A friend's wife left him for another relationship, and he has to establish a more distant yet respectful relationship to her and to his children, whom he sees less often. My mother is getting very old; I have to forget the many slights of childhood and make peace so we can both carry on our lives together. Each of the transitions in this second group seems to be less happy than the earlier ones, but we must face the shifts presented us just the same. How we respond to the significant choices we face determines the quality of our lives after transition. If we deny the changes and fight against them, we have a bad divorce, a bad parent-child relationship, a bad relationship with our aging parent.

If we accept the changes in the other person (my friend's ex-wife is now a distant friend; the woman's addicted son now needs her help in a new way), we have the opportunity to build a new and fruitful relationship that can enrich both our lives. All the transitions we go through as a result of the passages in other people's lives—both happy and sad ones—seem to be forced upon us. They are. That's life. A loved one starting to live with Alzheimer's and the relationship we build with that person is one of those transitions. We have the choice of making this change miserable for everyone; or we can make the best of it. We can do even better—we can improve all our lives by responding to and managing the transition positively.

The person who finds out he has Alzheimer's is the same person he was the day before. In the beginning he might become worried about the future—how is he going to live with this frightening illness? He needs a friend and information to understand what is going on and what the future is likely to hold. As he continues to live with Alzheimer's he changes even more—just as we all change as we age, but more dramatically. No matter what we go through, we need friends and partners with whom to build relationships. Building is the operant word. No matter what our relationship was to each other—husband/wife, parent/child, sister/brother, friend/friend—one thing is certain: that relationship will definitely not stay the same. A new one must be constructed.

The person living with Alzheimer's you used to love in one way—as your mother or father, your husband or wife, your sister or brother, and, in rare cases, your child—is turning into a new person whom you can embrace and enjoy. All happy change is tinged with sadness; all sad changes are tinged with joy. Sadness and joy are two sides of the same coin when you and the person you love find out you are living with Alzheimer's. It is essential for everyone's happiness, if not survival, that both people continue to see the good as well as the bad as the disease progresses and the relationship continues to change.

It is easy to say, "Forget the old person! Give up the old image!" But it is incredibly difficult to do. There are several reasons it is so hard and each has to be addressed if the transition is to be a positive one. The image a partner holds of the person she loves is of a person in whom she has invested a great deal of love and caring, a person who has shared many of life's other passages, and a partner with whom in some cases she has expected to grow old (as a spouse or sibling) or to enjoy later in life as they have enjoyed each other earlier (as a parent or child). "How can I just give all that up?" each of us asks ourselves.

The first answer is, you don't have to. The person living with Alzheimer's still has many of the experiences and characteristics that have made her who she has always been. She just can't draw on these life experiences and express them in the same way. What a partner has to give up is the unreal image he has in mind of the person he wishes the other would be. While she still has in herself all the past experiences of a life together, her future is no longer the one the partner dreamed of having. It is hard to give up the dreams each of us has had about our own future. Partners have to replace the fairy tale stories they have held on to for so long with new reality-based dreams.

There may be social pressures not to admit—and even to hide the fact—that the person has changed. Couples will have friends who know them as a couple and who expect them to be together when they come to visit. It is easier to set the stage for a shaky visit with friends, covering up for a husband's lapses of memory, than to admit he is a different person.

A third reason it is hard to give up the old image of a loved person is that we tend to define ourselves partly in terms of the other person. Our relationship to our spouse, parents, siblings, and our children form large parts of the definition of who we are, of how we see ourselves. We spend so much time engaged in trying to answer the question "Who am I?" that when we're forced to start again, it is a shock to the system. The image each of us holds on to is not of the other person, but of ourselves. To break this habit requires taking time with yourself to see and define who you are—without including the image of the other person as they were, or as you would like them to be.

Bill Keane, my colleague, friend, and mentor in matters dealing with Alzheimer's, who served for several years on the board of the National Alzheimer's Association, tells a moving story about his parents that indicates how aware the person living with Alzheimer's is of the need for acceptance of the transition into Alzheimer's. When his mother fell ill with Alzheimer's he cared for her personally for many years, eventually moving her to a nursing home where he visited her daily, bringing the cookies she liked, her favorite perfume, a hug, and a smile. He describes the wonderful loving relationship he developed with his mother while, on the other hand, she became increasingly estranged from his father—her husband—who loved his wife and had a difficult time accepting her illness. She must have been aware that Bill's father felt his life was over when he realized she had Alzheimer's disease, and she emotionally distanced herself from him. As Bill tells it, she knew deep down that her husband never accepted her for the person she had become. Bill says he knew his father felt this way because he "kept renewing Mom's driver's license until the end of her life." Somehow she knew this. A major reason for accepting—even embracing—the changes that come with living with Alzheimer's is that the person you love will know that you continue to love them.

BEGINNING A NEW RELATIONSHIP

A new relationship starts with letting go and embracing change. This is difficult and takes practice—practice paying attention, observing, and listening.

This is a study of human character, not a haphazard gathering of impressions or occasional thoughts. The partner of someone living with Alzheimer's who really wants to be able to build a positive relationship based on what he or she discovers, needs to approach this task seriously and carry it out rigorously.

Take these steps to discover the person within:

1. Keep a written log.
2. Take notes.
3. Record actual behavioral observations.
4. Write down "quotations" to which you might want to refer later.
5. Note the time of day and day of the week.
6. Describe the physical environment and social context of each observation.
7. Take digital photos of activities, interactions, and physical context.

The goal is both simple and incredibly complex—to discover the uniqueness of the person living with Alzheimer's.

The person's past likes and dislikes, and her experiences—successes and failures, achievements, hobbies, aptitudes, and dreams—are still there. But the past is now a context for better understanding the new person. Combining this knowledge with what you see, you should be able to discover the new person you are going to get to know.

Staying present to the person enables discovery of his present skills and aptitudes, not only those he used to have and you wish he still had. You discover those that may be reduced from earlier times such as certain cognitive ones; and those that may have improved, such as emotive and emotional knowledge. While the person you used to know was exceptional at multitasking, the new person is better at focusing on a particular person or task.

You also discover what makes her happy. She loves holding hands, walking in the garden, and shopping. She enjoys pets, children, and old movies—especially romantic ones.

You discover what makes him sad. He remembers his wife (your mother) with sadness because she passed away a few years ago, and he is sad when he thinks about the friends he lost in the war a long time ago. He is sad when you leave him after paying him a visit.

Based on your observations of both the person and yourself, you can start to build your new relationship. The new relationship has many dimensions and the following actions can help create a positive one.

- *The way you say hello.* Sit down next to her, hold her hand, look her in the eye, and say, "Hi, Mom, I'm your daughter Miriam, and I love talking with you about Oakland, where you were born." Don't just say "Hi, Mom" as you used to.

- *Topics of conversation.* Tell him about your day, and discuss what you know of his day. Talk about sports, politics, family, his past, your past together, the job he used to have, or just any subject that comes to mind. Don't sit quietly waiting for a topic of conversation to arise. It won't.

- *The rhythm of encounters/visits.* Start each visit excitedly talking about the things you did that day and slowly turn down the energy level until she walks you to the door. Or calmly chat the entire time you're there and then divert her attention to something else when you quietly slip away. Don't expect her to dictate the rhythm of the encounter.

- *The images you bring to communicate with him.* Bring photos, trophies from your childhood, news clippings from significant events in his life, a video of the family saying hello, or that day's newspaper to tell him about the world.

- *The props with which you surround the person.* Make sure there are familiar paintings on the wall and discuss them when you're with him. Make sure he has a bedspread he knows is his. It is a memory jogger. Don't buy new furnishings or clothes to make him feel good, as it might you. Make sure he has direct access to that easy chair he always sat in.

- *The way you arrange the house or the room.* Simplify the kitchen so it is least confusing and so that she can make a sandwich with no one else's help. Move the coffee table in the living room and put her favorite chair directly opposite the window so that she does not bump her knees getting to the chair, and so that she can see out easily when seated. Arrange lots of memory joggers around her bedroom.

- *The things you do together.* Create opportunities to do things together; don't wait for them to arise on their own. Take the initiative to walk in the garden together or down the street. Take the initiative to drive to an ice cream shop and share an ice cream cone. Go out to dinner.

- *The cultural events you attend.* Go regularly to the museum he was a member of. Buy tickets to the opera for him and you. What about the circus? Would he enjoy that? If you think he might, get tickets and have a good time. What about visiting the local historical society with pictures of the town when he was young?

- *The sequence of things you do together.* Decide how you are going to spend your time together. Don't leave it to chance. Plan a sequence, such as sitting together, then going out, driving around, stopping for a snack, and returning home. Or get his coat on right away, go out, and then sit for a while when you get back before you leave. Don't expect things to just happen by themselves.

- *The way you say good-bye.* Decide if you are going to explain to her when you leave where you are going and when you will be back. If so, be sure to describe these events simply. In a group setting, when you are going to leave, make sure she is involved in another activity with someone else before leaving. If you find this works well, time your leaving to coincide with something else going on that will interest her, then, if it makes you comfortable, prepare what you are going to take with you, pick it up, and say offhandedly "Bye, Mom" as you are at the door.

- *Leaving a record of your visit.* Decide what sort of trace you will leave of your visit. My colleague Cameron Camp suggests that if your mother used to have a Visitor Book in her house, you might put one in her room, one with a bright-colored cover. Every time you come to see her, write your name, the date and time, and a note about what you did together. If that feels too formal, put a large calendar on the wall and sign it each time you see her.

While some of these principles apply to all partners, each needs to be practiced differently by family members, professional-care partners, and others.

9

why changing yourself
is vital to effective
treatment

Medication is not a substitute for changing the things going on around the person or how caregivers respond to him.

—NANCY MACE AND PETER RABINS

BEING a full partner on the journey that is Alzheimer's requires more than merely watching others "treat" the illness. A full partner must also become part of her loved one's nonpharmacological treatment. Changing yourself is part of the treatment.

Partnering starts with building a new relationship on the foundation of the old one. A defining characteristic of the new relationship is that it will be mutually codependent. When the term "codependent" is applied to emotional bonds, it often refers to an excessive feeling of dependence one person has on another. The person feels that she "can't live without" the other. A person living with Alzheimer's actually does need other people, and does need her partner to remain at her highest quality of life. At the same time, the partner on the journey needs the person with Alzheimer's to be present to what the partner brings to the relationship.

Every individual recognizes others who are in need. This is likely a hardwired connection that the release of oxytocin awakens in the brain. The more sensitive to emotional expressions a person is—and people living with Alzheimer's are particularly sensitive thanks to their healthy amygdala—the more responsive he will be to other people's needs. A person living with Alzheimer's is a participant in every mutually caring relationship—if his partner knows how to open herself to being cared for.

The relationship you are likely to find is a yin and yang one in which both partners' needs and what they can give are intertwined. At the start of the journey, the interdependence can be developed as a contract between two people. The two can agree to give what they can to each other. As Alzheimer's progresses, planned exchanges become more difficult, and all you can do when this occurs is give of yourself to the other person. The amazing thing that often happens is that the person living with Alzheimer's finds that she needs to give as well—to figure out how to make you feel better, to express empathy with the moods that you express and that she recognizes, to tell you how much she loves you. She is responding with the hardwired part of her brain where a need to care for others is embedded.

Use every available trick and instinct in the relationship. Be vigilant—continually think about the effects of what you say and do in the relationship, both when you are together as well as apart.

- *Amygdala emotions.* Be sure to ask the person with Alzheimer's for expressions of emotions rather than cognitive data. Ask how they feel about a topic, not who was there a little while ago, or someone's name.
- *Memory joggers.* In conversation, bring up all the topics you have identified as jogging her memory. These may include a particular aspect of her life—her neighborhood or her job, her children or grandchildren, or particular life events. Whatever you do to trigger her access to memories plays a part in her treatment.
- *Visual props.* Photographs you share, mementos of special events, graduation certificates, military medals, a local team's baseball hat, anything three-dimensional that has meaning and that you can employ to generate interest or conversation is part of his treatment. Don't worry if there is a sad reaction to some of this. Enabling him to be present to his own memories and emotions is the gift and the goal.

- *Be the conversation generator yourself.* Be prepared to talk about your day, the kids, your work, the way you feel about a movie you saw, a trip you took recently. Don't expect the other person to draw on his memory bank of topics and recent experiences to generate conversation. If you have to carry the conversation as a monologue, carry it. To do this you may need to make and refer to a written list of topics you are going to cover, like a cue card.

A person who tries to implement all of the suggestions in this book might well collapse from exhaustion. To do everything oneself to maintain a relationship and provide meaning to another's life would take more time than there is in a day, and more energy than anyone has. It is essential, therefore, to take the things-to-do suggestions one at a time, and even to think of getting others to help carry them out.

THE CAREGIVING RESPONSIBILITY

Many partners feel they need to handle every situation by themselves. They believe that the personal relationship they have had for so long requires them to maintain this intimacy alone during the Alzheimer's journey. Thinking this way creates an unmanageable burden.

Whether the person living with Alzheimer's is parent, spouse, sister, or brother engaging him or her in life cannot be the sole responsibility of a single person. The title of one of the first books in this field, *The 36-Hour Day,* reflects the fact that when a person is the only one caring for another, he has to be so vigilant, and sleep so little, that each day feels half again as long as it really is. The person has to be half awake all night long. There is literally never any real rest. If you have let other members bow out of partnering without protecting yourself, ask yourself why you allowed this to happen. There are probably several good reasons.

One reason people—mostly spouses—become the sole care partners for their husbands or wives is the guilt they feel for abandoning them in an hour of need.

An Australian research project aimed at greater understanding of the perceptions and attitudes of family caregivers focused on twenty spouses of people who were in a nursing home. They were asked how they felt about their spouse being there. Ten people were there because of a nondementia condition like cancer. The other ten were living with dementia and were there because their spouse could no longer care for them at home. The feelings expressed by the first group included sadness and despair. Members of the second group, with a spouse in a nursing home because of Alzheimer's, all expressed a different emotion—guilt.

When the researchers probed further, they found that each spouse felt that going into a nursing home for cancer or a broken hip was natural and that if they were involved with the decision, they had done the right thing. The other group felt guilty, not because they could not do enough, but because they felt that breaking their marriage vows was wrong. They had promised to care for the person they married "until death do us part," and they felt that in not being able to take care of the spouse, they were breaking this promise. None of the ten husbands or wives in the second group could see the parallel between the destruction of an organ such as the liver, pancreas, skin, or lungs, and the destruction of another organ—the brain—in Alzheimer's disease. They saw cancer as a physical illness, and Alzheimer's as a mental illness that they should be able to care for at home. It is important to remind yourself that Alzheimer's is an organic illness of the brain, and that sharing care-partnering tasks with others is keeping a promise, not breaking it.

The same complex set of feelings comes into play when a person promised never to place the one they love "into a home." The "home" of olden days, the snake pit where older people disappeared and were never heard from again, may still exist somewhere. But today there are many wonderful places a man or woman with Alzheimer's can live, and where a spouse can be part of that person's life and treatment for the rest of their lives. Such a place is not the "home" about which the "never in a home" promise was made.

Once a decision is made that it is not only okay but even necessary to have other family members share the responsibility of partnering, a confrontation is inevitable. Conflict is likely to be part of any conversation with adult children about giving back to a parent—especially one they might not have had such an easy life with—and with close relatives living far away about needing their help. Families now are often spread around; a parent living in New York might have a son in California, a daughter in Paris, and another son in Montreal. When a mother calls her children, or an adult child calls her brother and sisters living far away to talk about changes taking place in their father's life, the physically distant relative may well say the differences in the person's behavior are not so great and that the person calling or e-mailing is being too extreme. "You can surely handle this yourself—we just visited and everything seemed okay," they may say. Family members can invent a myriad of excuses to avoid getting involved. Two major ones are the definition of the situation, and money.

- *The definition of the situation.* The only way to know what is really going on with a person living with Alzheimer's is to be there. No one can understand such a profound experience— both the good and the difficult—from a distance. If you make a visit with the person as normal, as comfortable, and as calm as possible, the visitors will assume everything is okay. If you let things get out of hand (incontinence, anger, distraction, agitation) visitors will think you are uncaring. It is imperative that every partner find a way to get other members of their family to understand what the situation really is like.

- *Money.* Throughout the progress of Alzheimer's and especially far into the illness, it costs a great deal to support the person and his partner. Just to find a little respite at home can require paying someone to sit with the person. There is the cost of taxis to replace the car that can't be driven, and the cost of handymen to fix things around the house that "he" used to fix himself. Everything gets more expensive. If a family decides that a special Alzheimer's program in an assisted-living residence would serve the person and his partner best, the costs are even greater, eating into the family nest egg. The farther away family members are from the situation, the less they understand that the real cost is the partner's sanity—a resource no one can afford to lose. Conflict around money between family members occurs frequently.

It is not easy to let strangers into one's life, but often the burden of not doing so is too great. Many professionals are ready to help, both at home and in communal settings.

- *The Alzheimer's Association.* Every local Alzheimer's Association has a help line where a real person who is often a volunteer with personal Alzheimer's experience—not an automated voice mail system—answers questions and directs callers to others who can help. The Alzheimer's Association also organizes and offers support groups in which people early in the illness as well as later on can share questions and worries with each other—sometimes in couples—and other partners can share their stories. There are often courses and conferences where both the person with Alzheimer's and his partner can gather new and helpful information.

- *Support groups for Alzheimer's partners.* Support groups offered at hospitals or other community settings provide more than mutual support—they allow partners to express frustrations, expectations, fears, joys, disappointments, and gifts with others who help them deal with what they are going through, plan next steps, and see the positive aspects of each situation.

- *Support groups for people living with an early stage of the illness in which partners participate.* At the beginning of this journey, both the person who has just learned he is going to live with Alzheimer's and his partner may be able to share their hopes and disappointments with others in a similar situation. If the support group leader is skilled and caring—and most are—participants learn, discuss, and eventually distance themselves enough from the immediate situation to see both the good and the bad, the joyous and the tragic, parts of it.

- *Geriatric care managers.* GCMs are professionals whose job it is to understand the family situation, and identify and provide needed help, especially if the partner or the person living with Alzheimer's is older. Help may be in the form of contact with an attorney who can arrange finances, links to an organization that provides suitable transportation to an event, or introduction to a communal living arrangement suited to the partner's and person's needs.

- *Medical professionals with expertise in Alzheimer's treatment.* For people just coming to grips with the fact that they or another is going to be living with Alzheimer's, and even if the person has been in this situation for some time, there are medical issues to deal with. A doctor with expertise in Alzheimer's treatment can help you understand the biology of the disease as well as help decide what, if any, medications to take. True medical experts can also advise on the best nonpharmacological treatments. In addition, medical tests can identify other illnesses with dementia symptoms, such as anemia, depression, and thyroid disease that are reversible. It is imperative to find out if such an illness is present and to deal with it immediately.

- *Health care professionals with expertise in Alzheimer's treatment.* Other health professionals like psychiatrists, nurses, or a neurologist may be able to help in the same way—as long as they have special and broad knowledge of Alzheimer's disease, its dynamics, and available nonpharmacological and pharmacological treatments.

- *Health care professionals in communal settings.* Even if there is no plan to move to a communal setting like an assisted-living residence or a nursing home, health and other professionals working at such a place might be able to listen and perhaps offer advice.

COMMUNAL RESOURCES AND RESIDENTIAL TREATMENT PROGRAMS

Communal resources and residential options may be helpful at some time during the progress of the illness to partners and people living with Alzheimer's. Information about such living situations is vital once partners realize they cannot do everything themselves and that trying to do so is stressful and disruptive for the care partner as well as for the person living with Alzheimer's. The range of communal resources and settings follows a continuum, from at home to institutional care.

This continuum does not necessarily reflect the progression of the disease. A person might never need a nursing home, or might move to a nursing home temporarily before finding a suitable assisted-living residence. Hospitals may serve a certain purpose early in the illness. Day programs may never be utilized, or they may be regularly employed to provide the partner with daily respite. Special assisted-living programs for those with Alzheimer's may be employed as a residential option early in the illness and throughout the person's life. Clearly, hospice is an optional end of life service.

Even if the person and her partner are not planning to take advantage of such options, everyone involved needs to know which services and settings are available and what each provides. Remember, when the partner takes care of herself, the person living with Alzheimer's does better as well.

The range of community services includes:

Home care and home health services. People living at home who need help getting things done can arrange for others to come into their homes and help them in many ways. This can be done informally by hiring individual helpers or through service agencies. A geriatric-care manager might be engaged to arrange these services. For help with daily tasks that have just become too difficult, like shopping, making meals, and cleaning up, home-care assistants can do the job. If the help includes assistance with health-related matters—such as dressing a wound or administering certain pills— a home health aide is called for. If the person for whom this arrangement is made is living with Alzheimer's, it is important that the person helping has specific training in behaviors related to the illness, in related symptoms, as well as in nonpharmacological treatment options. The helper must be prepared and know what to do when the person living with Alzheimer's says she does not want strangers in her house and "fires" the helper as soon as she arrives. If the helper is trained to handle such situations, she will know how to make friends and stay on the job. If a helper is hired to stay overnight, he must be prepared to stay up and not complain that he has two jobs and needs his sleep. Such help can provide needed respite for a person living with someone who has Alzheimer's disease, but a helper who does not know how to do his job provides little respite.

Social and medical day programs. People who live and sleep at home may also spend part of their day in a safe place away from home where they become involved in activities of all sorts and at the same time receive a healthy lunch. A partner in need of time off who wants the person to be safe and engaged may be the one making the decision, or both people may decide together. The services that day programs offer may include transportation to and from a center, and may focus on social or medical issues. Social programs include activities much of the day. Medical day programs include such services as reminders to take medications, help with taking medications, as well as physical or other rehabilitation services. An activity program and help with daily living activities are also usually included in medical day programs so the person enjoys the time he spends there.

Special assisted-living programs. Some people may decide that living in a residential group community serves their needs best.

It is essential to avoid confusing mainstream assisted living with special programs for people living with Alzheimer's. These programs tend to have designed environments with safe gardens, staff trained to talk to and provide support to people living with Alzheimer's, and activities planned to engage people living with Alzheimer's through every stage of the illness. Special assisted-living programs like these also tend to encourage family members to remain a central part of their loved one's lives—coming and going as often as and whenever they like.

Nursing home special care units. When people have physical needs that require twenty-four-hour a day nursing or just feel they want the sense of security that twenty-four-hour on-site nursing may provide, they can move into a nursing home. Most nursing homes, or at least any nursing home suitable for a person living with Alzheimer's, have special-care units, or SCUs, for people with Alzheimer's. Merely having an Alzheimer's diagnosis is not usually a reason for living in a nursing home—also called an SNF, or skilled nursing facility. And not every SCU is the same—the quality of such places varies greatly. "Wards" that distinguish themselves from other units by having their doors locked and alarmed but have no specially trained staff or programs are sometimes called SCUs, but really are not. Higher-quality SCUs have trained staff and special programs and also tend to have some of the same residential features that special assisted-living programs have for people with Alzheimer's. It is important to carefully assess the quality of the SCU being selected, if this is the option best suited to the person and the family.

Hospitals. Especially in emergency situations, a hospital may be the best place to go for help. A person with Alzheimer's who lives alone at home and progresses in the disease without others being aware may end up with an emergency—an accident, lack of nutrition, or a fall. Hospitals are likely to be the best place to go for help when this occurs. It is important to be certain that hospital staff know that their patient is living with Alzheimer's. They need to be told this when the person arrives so that they can treat him with special care and allow a partner or friend to stay with him throughout the hospital stay, to relieve anxiety, explain what the patient may be trying to say, and avoid misunderstandings. And they need the Alzheimer's training to know how to provide this care.

Hospice programs. At the end of life there are many people available to help the person and the family go through this passage. When this option is chosen it is essential to engage a program that includes staff specially trained to respond to people who have been living with Alzheimer's.

A COMMON PHILOSOPHY OF CARE

A family hiring a nanny to take care of children full-time makes sure to interview her about her child-rearing attitudes. Does she believe in lots of television, or in getting children involved in games? In good weather would she expect to stay indoors or go outdoors with the children? What is her attitude toward discipline? What would she do if a child fell down and hurt his knee? Parents make sure that her approach mirrors theirs so that when they are away they can be generally certain that the same messages that they would give are being given to the children.

The same holds true for people living with Alzheimer's, and their partners or families who might share partnering with professionals. There are several steps in doing this.

- *Figure out what you want.* In the beginning of the illness the person living with Alzheimer's needs to share with her partners what her philosophy is about her own care when she may eventually need it. It is important that this be done before reaching out to a professional. Don't react to another's definition of which path to follow. Discuss and decide with your partner and for yourself the kind of life you would like to have. Do the necessary research—read, visit, go to lectures, talk to people, and take part in Alzheimer's Association early-stage support groups. Then decide.

- *Insist on working only with professionals who share your approach.* There are many different approaches to this illness, all of which can be legitimate. Don't let someone tell you what to believe just because they have more experience and more degrees. If the professional in whose presence you find yourself insists on talking you out of what you believe, walk away and find another.

- *Make agreements with your partner and with professionals about treatment and end of life.* Treatment approaches and end-of-life decisions need to be consensual.

- *Treatment.* This book presents a particular approach toward treatment of the illness and toward people living with Alzheimer's disease. The approach includes both nonpharmacological interventions such as environment, communication, and activities, as well as selective medications balanced in a total coordinated treatment. Nonpharmacological modalities are suggested first, and medications are employed only when nonpharmacological ones do not have the expected symptom-reducing effects. Family and partners need to insist on finding professionals who share their approach—whether the one I provide in this book or another.

- *End-of-life decisions.* This book does not take a position on the moral and ethical character of any end-of-life decisions that a family, spouse, or child should take in case the person living with Alzheimer's is dying. Whatever decisions are made must include the person's own beliefs. Professionals involved must respect and share that point of view.

- *Insist on specialty training.* Alzheimer's is not the same as old age. It is a disease that affects certain people when they get older, and the older we get, the higher the chance of living with the disease and exhibiting its symptoms. When choosing a doctor for advice, diagnosis, and involvement in treatment, pharmacological or nonpharmacological, be sure that he or she has special training in dementia and Alzheimer's. Finding specialists to work with who share the same philosophy and approach to life, illness, and death avoids great pain and frustration for the person living with Alzheimer's and for family members and partners.

    If a community-based program fits into the treatment picture—home care, day program, assisted living, nursing home, hospital, or hospice—insist on knowing how and where the professionals and care partners were trained to deal with people living with Alzheimer's. Don't ask just about how long they studied; ask what they learned. Everyone has the right to ask such questions, as well as the responsibility. Don't let anyone avoid answering questions by telling you that you wouldn't understand the specifics of the training program.

Every service available to elders has a parallel service available to people living with Alzheimer's. There are home-care services with aides trained to communicate with people living with Alzheimer's. The same is true for day and hospice programs. It is important for care partners to share their burden with those who understand the disease and to rely on programs and settings formulated to respond to the needs of people living with Alzheimer's.

Whether in an assisted-living residence or a nursing home, Alzheimer's-friendly and capable programs make a great difference to residents' quality of life. The centers will have special design features, such as access to a therapeutic garden, and will have staff members who want to work there because they have a natural empathy with elders living with Alzheimer's.

In quality programs for people living with Alzheimer's, basic care characteristics ought not to be overlooked.

- *High-quality basic health care.* A place that is high quality for someone suffering from any illness has to treat her basic health care needs well. Medications when prescribed need to be taken at the right time and in the right dose. If a person is likely to fall, appropriate precautions need to be taken and the right procedures followed to avoid additional damage. Healthy meals, a well-maintained environment, and engaging and meaningful activities are all part of quality health care. Of course, physical problems must be diagnosed and treated without relying on the person living with Alzheimer's to verbally describe the symptoms.

- *Partner participation.* Partners know more about the person living with Alzheimer's than anyone else. Family members know his history and, if they have developed a new relationship with him, they know him at the moment better than anyone else as well. Staff in high-quality settings recognize this and include partners in treatment decisions and everyday life. Not only are partners allowed to participate in bringing their personal knowledge to health care, they are invited to do so. Higher-quality programs will have formal as well as informal mechanisms to achieve this.

- *Being part of the "treated" not only the "treatment."* The effects of Alzheimer's are part of every partner's life, as is the case with every chronic illness and disability. Partners and other family members are affected emotionally, and feel nervous, upset, angry, or unreasonable throughout the illness. Staff in a good program will take care of the partner and welcome her as a care partner even if she is upset and "difficult" at times. Staff will understand what partners can't do as well as what they can do, and will help them to do their best.

It is not enough that those caring for and treating a parent or spouse in a community setting know about Alzheimer's disease and how it affects the person. People working together need to understand how to communicate—in bad times as well as good. This means dealing with emergencies, conflict, trust, and other important issues that affect health outcomes. Special teamwork training can get this process moving in the right direction. At Hearthstone, we include teamwork training for all staff so that the best possible decision for residents is made as often as possible.

If there is one single thing to look for in selecting a group or organization to turn to for help, it is how compassionate it is. When my friend and colleague Robin Orr, an expert in health care design and culture, learned she had cancer she found her-self in the grips of the health care system. After more than a year of multiple radiation and chemotherapy sessions, she decided to lecture about what she found most lacking in her treatment and care: compassion. Since she received her first speaking request on the topic of compassion, we have been working together to identify what a compassionate organization would look like. How would a highly compassionate organization differ from a less compassionate one? Some of the ideas we've explored are having staff members treated with the same dignity and respect as pa-tients, that each person would be cared for in body, mind, and spirit, that each person's lifestyle would be accommodated, and that fun and joy would be part of the culture. Our commitment is to make compassion the "visible" ingredient in health and healing. However, if you name it—"come to our compassionate assisted-living program for people living with Alzheimer's"—you have already lost some of the compassion you are looking for. In her lectures worldwide, Robin is searching for indicators of compassion in health and healing. As you search for a place for yourself and the person you love living with Alzheimer's, you too can look for these indicators.

Compassion also plays a significant role in taking care of yourself. Finding ways to ease your workload and emotional burden indirectly does not replace taking care of yourself directly. At some point in this journey you will definitely have to face this fact.

TAKING CARE OF YOURSELF

Those who care for people living with Alzheimer's tend not to take care of themselves. They tend to get sick more often and for longer periods than the people they care for.

In Western philosophy, the term *compassion* refers to feelings a person has about the plight or problems of others. The *Cambridge Dictionary of American English,* for example, defines *compassion* as: "a strong feeling of sympathy and sadness for other people's suffering or bad luck and a desire to help."

The Bible employs the word in both the Old Testament and

the New Testament: "He being full of compassion, forgave their iniquity" (Psalms 78:38); "His father . . . had compassion, and ran, and fell on his neck, and kissed him" (Luke 15:20).

A compassionate person feels for others in need and in trouble. Compassion for the other in the extreme can lead the compassionate person to give of herself until she gets sick. Living with Alzheimer's is both constant and engaging, often eliciting extreme compassion.

The concept of compassion in Buddhist philosophy refers to similar feelings of understanding and sympathy. But there is a difference. Buddhist compassion describes feelings a person has for all beings—including himself. Compassion of this sort—for all sentient beings—would naturally lead a person to take care of himself, not to sacrifice himself for another—it just doesn't make sense.

If the partner of someone living with Alzheimer's gets sick, the person living with Alzheimer's suffers. Throughout the passage of the illness, awareness that another person is there for him keeps the man or women with Alzheimer's going, keeps his spirits high. In early phases, people feel their partners helping them stay connected to life and society. At later stages, a partner may not feel the person with Alzheimer's knows he is there or even remembers who he is. This is most unlikely. She may not be able to recall a name precisely, but her amygdala makes sure she knows and feels the other's love and concern. A person's spouse, child, sibling, and friend are always emotionally important to them—throughout their lives with Alzheimer's.

Here are some key pieces of advice for partners when things get difficult:

- Live within your own capabilities and limits.
- Don't push the limits as far as they will go.
- Establish your own life and rhythm.
- Establish a lifeline or two.
- Learn to say, "Please help me."
- Learn to give up.

Live within your own capabilities and limits. How old are you? How is your health? How much can you endure? How many others are you taking care of—a husband, children, another parent? Do you have a job in which you have to perform up to a certain standard? Answers to such questions determine how much caregiving and treatment a partner can take on.

Your health depends on living within the limits of your capability. None of us likes to admit that we are mortal, fallible, and human or that we can't do something we want to do. But if we don't live within the limitations we have at this time in our lives, the person living with Alzheimer's suffers as well.

Don't push the limits as far as they can go. When asked when they are going to take action—seek help, find another housing arrangement, attend a support group—many partners say, "It's not bad enough *yet*." Not bad enough yet! Think about what this means. It means that the partner's measure of when to act is the degree of discomfort, suffering, and pain she can endure without collapsing or getting sick. It is essential for each partner's health, and thus the relationship of mutual help and compassion between the two, that this way of thinking be abandoned. The measure of when to act is when it is best for the relationship— which means when it is best for both the person living with Alzheimer's and the partner. The longer people hold out before taking action, the longer is the period of "yet"—as in "It's not bad enough yet"—and the higher the likelihood that something catastrophic may occur such as a fall or a fire, and the greater the chance that the partner may fall ill.

Establish your own life and rhythm. As the person continues to progress into Alzheimer's, she will have a new life and become a new person. Partners need to establish their own new life as well. That is the only way partners stay healthy, even when the person remains central to a partner's life forever.

Establishing a new life entails:

- *New skills.* Learn how to keep a schedule, perhaps using a handheld personal planner.
- *New hobbies.* Didn't you always want to learn to play golf?

- *New pleasures.* Didn't you always want to go swimming every morning and go to the opera once a month?
- *Trips you always wanted to take.* Go on a cruise with an old friend.
- *New friends.* How about new friends to whom present friends might introduce you?
- *A new schedule.* Perhaps you can plan to be with the person living with Alzheimer's every afternoon and keep mornings and evenings for yourself.

Establish a lifeline or two. Being a partner of someone living with Alzheimer's is trying, no matter how positive partners may feel about it. And it becomes more trying as the disease progresses. There will be times when you will despair. There will be times when you don't want to get up in the morning. At times like this you need to have friends or professional helpers who are lifelines you can rely on.

- *Whom can you "vent" to?* To whom can you pour out your heart with all its anguish and fear? To whom can you rail against your fate and the fate of the person living with Alzheimer's whom you love? To whom can you shout the "terrible" feelings you have? You need to identify that person, and make sure she or he understands something about the disease as well as how feeling helpless does not mean giving up.

- *Find a formal support group of people dealing with similar issues.* It is not enough to be in a group of people who are at the same stage you are. It is better if there are people further along the journey who can tell you something about what you can expect, and others further behind for whom you can lead the way. In this way you can be a person in need, a person getting help, and a person helping others all at the same time.

At least as important as the support group's membership is its facilitator. Attend a support group led by a social worker, a program administrator, a trained care partner, or anyone else you like and trust. The facilitator or leader is the person who orchestrates the mix of emotional learning and cognitive learning the group embraces. He or she knows when to let people express themselves, and when too much expression may hurt others. The facilitator is the person who knows where to find additional resources—people and written material—that may help in participants' journeys, and knows which of these is of high quality. If you don't like the leader, find another group you feel is more sympathetic to your concerns and needs.

Learn to say, "Please help me." One of the gifts of Alzheimer's is that the act of caring for another teaches us to be aware of our own frailties and limits. A related gift is that we learn that we need others, and that they need us. In order to take care of ourselves, we all need to learn to say, "Please help me."

Learn to give up. In this journey there is always a point when you can't go further—at least at that moment. You have to learn to do what you can do, and learn to give up and drop it when the tasks at hand are overwhelming. This eloquent secular paraphrase of Reinhold Niebuhr's well-known "serenity" prayer says it all:

Know yourself well enough to do what you can, accept what you can't, and avoid deceiving yourself into believing that you can achieve the impossible.

10

THE GIFTS OF
ALZHEIMER'S

insights gained
from learning to give
and receive

Feelings form the base for what humans have described for millennia as the
human soul or spirit.   —ANTONIO R. DAMASIO

⌘ THERE is life after an Alzheimer's diagnosis, and there is life
for the partner of someone living with Alzheimer's disease. The
term "Alzheimer's" brings to mind for many a false image of a
sick, old, bedridden person whose mind wanders, who forgets
the names of friends and family, and who is rapidly becoming a
nonperson. This extreme mental picture develops because the
media frequently presents this image and because those who
fund-raise for cure research find that such an image stirs people's
hearts—as well as their pocketbooks. The picture of someone
living with the illness attending a concert or enjoying a museum

does not pull on the heartstrings of potential donors. The image of a sick dependent old person also develops because living with Alzheimer's frightens us. It reminds us that we too are vulnerable to the ravages of time and age.

Of course this picture is mostly untrue—unless the ends of all our lives are to be pictured, living with or without Alzheimer's. People with Alzheimer's live most of their lives with bodies at least as healthy as those of others their age—and minds that work, although stressed more by everyday situations than is true for many others. So far this book has described how engaging people living with Alzheimer's can awaken them and their partners.

But there is more that can be positive in a life with Alzheimer's. Being present to someone living with the illness teaches profound, usually unspoken, and often surprising lessons to those open to change. For them it is as if the relationships foster and unwrap special personal "gifts" in the developing relationship. In relationship with people living with Alzheimer's, we learn a great deal both about them and about ourselves.

Ellen Pall, writing in *The New York Times* (December 25, 2005), describes eloquently how her relationship with her father as he developed Alzheimer's enhanced her view of the world.

While her father moved further into Alzheimer's, he focused more and more on trees. He would point at trees he saw and say, "Look." And Ellen, without knowing quite what he meant, would indeed get behind him to see the trees from his vantage point and "look."

When she and her siblings were young, her father was kind and attentive, playing guitar and singing folk songs to them before they went to sleep. After Ellen's mother died, when she was only seven, he became distant and paid more attention to his work. "All these years he and I were not close," she writes. "I desperately wished to be," she continues, "but I saw him as cold and removed, uninterested in personal life . . . I would never have said we were close—until he got Alzheimer's."

Ellen began to feel she had received the gift of relationship with her father only after he had lived with Alzheimer's for several years. She brought him music—"a recording of a rhapsodic Georges Enesco composition was 'the most beautiful music' he had ever heard"—and started a new relationship. He showed wonder, surprise, and pleasure whenever he saw her, and was extremely kind, sharing his food when she visited. Ellen ends her story describing the effect her father's joy in trees had on her.

Now my father is dead, my mother is dead, and I am next in line. . . . In the summer, when I see trees lighted by the sun, moving in the wind, I am amazed at their beauty. Some of their leaves wink like coins, some wave like hands. Sometimes a whole branch sighs and bows, like a courtier. Look. Look!

Seeing the world through her father's eyes, Ellen established a new relationship with him. It reflected the way they loved each other when she was young. Many parents and children never achieve this; Ellen did through Alzheimer's. The awe and joy in Ellen's new view of trees was a true gift.

"The Gifts of Alzheimer's" is what I call a type of discussion to which I regularly invite family members and partners. No one in such a group embraces the disease saying, "I am so happy my wife [or mother or sister] is living with Alzheimer's." All say that if there were any way to return to the time before Alzheimer's entered their lives, they would jump at the chance. But there isn't.

The subject of our discussions is the way each of us has "improved" as human beings as a result of the relationship we have built with our loved ones over time. These are the gifts we receive.

At the start of each Gifts of Alzheimer's discussion I describe my own experience over the past ten to fifteen years spent with the people we care for at Hearthstone—which includes the loved ones of those in the group. I tell them:

I used to be angrier. After my divorce, angry that my kids were not with me more, I took it out on my family, my children, and my stepchildren. I was impatient, always on the move, seldom present to what others were experiencing at the moment. I usually focused on my own experiences, not others'. To take advantage of life and live it to its fullest I pushed the limits of every relationship.

As I increasingly spent time with people living with Alzheimer's, I realized that anger and impatience worked against me. If I was impatient with someone living with Alzheimer's, they would react by withdrawing. If I was angry about anything at all, they would get angry back or at least become anxious and agitated. On the other hand, being present to each person I was with led to more profound friendships and relationships than when I thought I was the center of the world. Over the years I have transferred these lessons to my own family. I have a loving relationship with my wife and all my children, and just "being" with both friends and strangers is extremely rewarding. The gifts I have received from all the people living with Alzheimer's I have known and know today are the gifts of patience, nonanger, and the joy of being present with others—just to be with another person in their own space with whoever they are at the moment.

Many people have joined me to explore gifts they have received from the people they love who are living with Alzheimer's. The following are their personal *gifts of Alzheimer's* stories.

The gift of emotional openness to others. "My mother is exquisitely open emotionally to me and to those around her. When I am happy or sad, she often understands how I feel sooner than others do and always responds with more empathy and compassion. I know she loves me and I am learning from her to be more open and loving myself."

The gift of cherishing memories. "With gentle reminders, my father recalls many memories of childhood, family, and friends. These seem timeless and appear not to be fading. The more I am with him the more I cherish these things in my own life and the more enriched I am. A smile from him and his hand closed on mine express this awareness as eloquently as a long speech would."

The gift of having a sense of humor. "Caring for my mother with Alzheimer's I have to laugh sometimes at the things that happen and at things she says. Now I can laugh at situations in the rest of my life that otherwise used to drive me up the wall."

The gift of accepting help. "I always thought I had to do everything myself, that I had to do all the caring. Now I can accept the help of others more. It is a blessing to be relieved of all the pressure I felt—all the responsibility."

The gift of taking care of myself. "I always thought that I needed to do everything for everybody. Now I realize that if I don't take care of myself, I won't be able to help my mother. I feel good taking care of myself now—just for its own sake."

The gift of recognizing the importance of home and hearth. "My father recognizes the value of where he is. He is surrounded by his own possessions—reminders of his past—that carry with them the joys and sorrows of his life. The more I get to know him again and realize the importance of his home to him, the more I value the friendliness of others, of sharing food, of having a place of my own."

The gift of life stories. "My mother can often tell better stories than other old people I know. She has an active imagination and deep memories of places and times from her past. She loves an appreciative audience. I hone my skills at storytelling the more I realize that this is a skill that will continually increase throughout my life, no matter what happens to me."

The gift of patience. "Whenever I try to speed things up when I am with my father I become aware that life has its own pace and that there is little I can do to speed it up or slow it down. He just tells me bluntly to relax, or he gets upset. Every time I am with my father, I develop more patience and understanding. My lack of patience becomes abundantly clear."

The gift of enjoying the moment. "My mother is perpetually in the moment. Whenever we are together, I am given the cherished gift of being there with her at that moment. Any regrets about the past I might have, or hopes and fears about the future, have little place in our relationship at that moment. The feeling of being present to life lingers on long after we have been together."

The gift of self-awareness. "Every expression and every movement of mine counts when I am with my mother and her friends. They notice everything around them and are exquisitely sensitive to nuance and detail. I have learned from her how important everything I do is to others. When I visit my mother, I am aware of how much she enjoys the first hug I give her—no words, just her soft and welcoming smile."

The gift of seeing others for who they are. "My mother and her friends have only themselves and their experiences. While they may still have certain skills or even money, those achievements and possessions pale in the light of who they are. When we are together, their smiles, their tenderness, their sensibilities— their basic human instincts—become the person I relate to—not their possessions."

The gift of disappearing problems. "My mother gets upset when she senses others are coping with unresolved problems. Whenever I drive to see my mother I prepare myself by emptying my mind of daily problems, no matter how immediate they may be. This is a skill I have only mastered since Mom has been living with Alzheimer's. It is not fair to bring these problems into encounters with her because she is so sensitive to my every mood. Even when I arrive for a visit with problems unresolved, by the time I leave my mind is clear and at peace—at least for the time being. Now I do the same things with my friends and family."

The gift of the importance of family. "Even though I am only thirty years old, contact with my friend living with Alzheimer's has made me realize how fragile and transitory life is. Now, even more than earlier in my life, I cherish the time I spend with my parents—no matter how difficult those relationships might be."

The gift of realizing that Plato was right. "Most of my adult life I thought I knew what things were—what was real and what was not. As my father developed Alzheimer's, I remembered my college philosophy class in which we studied the writings of the Greek philosopher Plato. One of these was the *Meno.* In it, Plato describes life as a cave at the center of which is a fire that casts shadows on the wall of people chained there. Reality is different to everyone because each person sees different shadows on the wall. People didn't see either the fire or themselves, only ever-changing shadows. Now I realize reality is like that. My father sees the shadows one way, and I see them another. And we're both right."

The gift of being prepared. "I never knew how much being prepared could help others and could help me. When Mom first started living with Alzheimer's I had trouble helping her get dressed. She would always get upset. Last week I had all her clothes laid out for her before she came into the room. It was a lot easier this time. It's a lesson for life."

The gift of knowing my work is "good" work. "When I massage these clients they have a big smile. I give them the gift of touch; in return they give me the gift of value—we're both getting something out of the massage. My own life has more value—you appreciate your own life more."

The gift of going with the flow. "With my husband I learned how just to be appropriate and to say the right thing. I learned I can only do what I can do—no more. So what if I can't go to a show or an event I wanted to attend. I greet each morning without plans. I just go with the flow—something I've never before been able to do."

The gift of coping with the complicated. "Nothing is simple with Alzheimer's. It's all just complicated. I've learned over time that I can handle it. I can handle all sorts of complicated things in the rest of my life too that I hadn't been able to handle."

The gift of keeping going. "When my husband was diagnosed a few years ago, I decided we're just going to keep going. Last month we took a boat ride to Nova Scotia. We play golf each week. We've been happily married for forty-two years. Every day I just try to make life as happy as it has always been—and it works."

The gift of greater insight. "Alzheimer's has opened a window into a part of my mother that was mostly guarded in the past. Now she is able for the first time to show the more affectionate part of her nature. There is less conflict between us now. I feel I can be more affectionate toward her. I have become more open not only to her, but to my family and friends as well."

The gift of giving. "It was always hard to please my father—no matter how hard I tried. Now he has 'the smile of the moment that means everything.' Now I always know when he is happy with something I have done for him, and I am able to give more freely of myself."

The gift of community. "When I come to visit my mother it's fun because all the people here respond so gleefully to me. Each person in this community has unique characteristics. It's wonderful for me and for my mother."

The gift of my own humanness. "I have learned to let go of my own reality—of thinking that 'my own home' is special and that my view of what is beautiful is the right view. No! It's their beauty that's important. People with Alzheimer's don't care about you as an individual. They don't ask for your résumé. All they want is a smile and a kind, warm look. They very quickly notice insincerity. Your humanness is all that matters."

The gift of emotional ties. "With people living with Alzheimer's you have a strong feeling of doing what *has* to be done to make their lives better. It's not a matter of thinking about what to do, or figuring out what's needed. You just know. It's so immediate. Rather than having emotional baggage, you find you have emotional ties."

The gift of listening. "People just want to be listened to. It's as if you're called out of a tense meeting for a phone call as opposed to having your cell phone go off in the meeting. It gives you a chance for energetic cleansing, recentering of your chi [vital energy]. You can regroup your thoughts and energy and reenter the meeting with a better attitude. That's what it's like being with my mother. She listens so well, and I listen to her so well. The result for me is that I feel energetically cleansed."

The gift of accepting death. "We always want to 'fix' everything, and yet there are certain things we can never fix. The true gift I have learned to give my mother is the strength to face her upcoming death. By accepting her for who she is, by my not feeling fear and alarm, she is at peace—and so am I."

The gift of growing up. "In order for me to cope with this disease and to learn new ways of being with my mother, I had to grow first, emotionally, spiritually, and mentally. From this growth I have gained hope—hope and belief that I have a chance of growing up someday."

The gift of "we." "It's hard to make it an 'I' when I am with my mother. If I am not connected to her when we are together, we lose each other. She is centered if I am centered. I have to give up the 'I' and become the 'we' with her—it's like the yin and yang symbol of Oriental philosophy. Except that instead of yin and yang, the connection is between the 'I' and 'You.'"

The gift of a kinder world. "My father shows more emotion now than he used to. He sees the world differently—not as competitive and not as possessive. I am learning to see it that way too."

The gift of nurture. "I never had children, so taking care of someone is new. It put me in a different role than I had experienced. Helping my mother helped me. I can nurture her. I used to think she knows better, no matter what the situation. I let go of my expectations of who and what she was before, and accept who she is now. I gave up thinking, 'She knows better.' It's no longer me, me, me in my life."

The gift of realizing life is precious. "Every day that I come to work, I learn so much from all these people living with Alzheimer's. I have twenty grandmothers now. Every day, I touch someone on a certain level. I see someone gaining ground in how to do something—even a simple task. When I come to work I could be in the best mood, or the worst. Now I live in the moment. I realize that no matter how lost a person may seem, there's still a person there. I call my own grandmother more often now. I see how precious she is. Even though I'm only twenty-three, I have learned that life is precious, and not seeing that is dumb."

The gift of capability. "When my mother got ill I found myself being very responsible and necessary. The sense of being needed was and is still very intense. I had a tremendous sense of obligation and duty. And I found out something else about myself. I never thought I could toilet my mother or clean her up after she was incontinent during the night. I learned I was personally capable of so much more than I thought I was."

The gift of revisiting. "Since my mother started living with

Alzheimer's I revisit old things and experiences in new ways. I am more balanced about them, more tolerant, more understanding. It is somewhat cyclical, looking at the past this way, but I get a smile from it."

The gift of taking risks. "Every so often my dad says, 'Kill me.' But every day they learn something new about the disease. I take more and more risks every day as a result of my dad's illness. I am glad to be alive now."

The gift of understanding basic truth. "It's actually very easy to understand people. I don't understand everything all the time, but my dad seems to. He's right there in the present. Last week my husband, who is very nervous, and my dad were lying on the bed and we had a lot of laughs. My husband told us he was worried about something he had forgotten to do. My dad said, "That's okay, that's what I do half the time around here." We were talking about the quality of the caregivers here. My dad said, "They have a good team here. Well, there are times you wish you were someplace else. But that's true anywhere." We all laughed at the basic truth of my dad's way of seeing the world."

The gift of valuing others. "I never thought I'd be taking care of my parents. I never thought I'd be changing my mother's clothes. I have had to develop a lot of patience, scheduling taking care of my parents along with taking care of my four kids. What I have gained is appreciating the value of others in my life."

The gift of the Zen mind. "My relationship with my father

has become incredibly direct. The illness has led to our narrowing things down—to a state of grace, to the Zen mind. Whereas before we might have analyzed everything and even fought about how we saw things, now it's just about 'Ow, it hurts!' and 'Oh.' "

The gift of control. "I'm grateful that my father and I have grown in our relationship. He is a new person. That 'old' person of my childhood wasn't so easy. He always had to be in control, and I distanced myself. Now he feels good that I am in control, and so do I."

The gift of conversation. "Whenever I realize how little I talked to my dad in my life, and that I can no longer have those conversations, I appreciate conversations more. I think about my friends and say appreciatively to myself, 'Oh my God, I can have a conversation with you!' It makes me want to talk more—to call up friends I haven't talked to for a while."

The gift of giving and of giving up. "Before my mother lived in this special place, there was such a dependency on the amount of support that I needed to give. Now that I don't have to provide that support I have inner peace, knowing that her basic needs are being met in a thoughtful way. This has released me to be ha-ha! hee-hee! with her. It's amazing how much you get by giving up. But you know, even though it was a lot of responsibility, I kinda miss it."

The gift of quality time. "I have gained a better sense of time in my own life. When you see them—the people with Alzheimer's who live here—you realize that time really is fleeting. You really know what quality time is."

The gift of kids coming to visit. "My kids were always afraid of visiting their grandfather. They didn't know how to deal with his illness. One thing that is so helpful for them, that is a real eye-opener, is the warmth that staff and families exhibit toward my father and everyone here. Seeing this has made them much more willing to come visit."

In sum, people living with Alzheimer's teach us to have open hearts and minds and to become better people. What we learn—the gifts we receive—helps us not only in those relationships, but also in all the relationships in our lives.

11

BEING IN THE PRESENT MOMENT

a mindfulness meditation

Be happy in the moment, that's enough. Each moment is all we need, not more. —MOTHER TERESA

GROUPS of neuroscientists have been meeting every few years for over a decade with the Dalai Lama at his retreat in Dharamsala, India, to explore the relationship between Western science and Eastern Buddhist philosophy. Of particular interest to them are the questions: how do emotions affect health, and can mindfulness meditation positively affect our immune system? In answering these questions, the work of Jon Kabat-Zinn, a neuroscientist and clinician who has developed an approach to health that focuses on the meditative practice called *mindfulness,* stands out. Kabat-Zinn's approach and the clinical practice that he established in the Stress Reduction Clinic at the University of Massachusetts Medical Center in Worcester, Massachusetts, has continued to grow in importance as others realize its positive impacts on health. As the psychologist and writer Daniel Goleman said, "Stripped of its religious context, mindfulness meditation is simply learning to have an open and accepting attitude toward whatever arises in one's mind. This very simplicity makes it useful as a stress-reduction technique."

Thich Nhat Hanh, a Zen Buddhist monk and teacher, employs a technique of guided meditation to help people be mindful in everyday life. Thich Nhat Hanh's approach uses a set of organized phrases based on critical issues in people's lives to focus their attention. Reciting these phrases silently to themselves as they quietly breathe in and out while meditating, helps them deal with the stress and cacophony of everyday life.

A line and a point represent two ways of experiencing the passing of time. The line of time that most of us experience comprises the past about which we hold many "what if" regrets, the present that is always fleeting—we never have "enough" time—and the future that we worry about because we can't predict which of the infinite alternative things that might happen will actually occur. We believe that a clearer vision of the future would help us make better decisions in the present moment.

THE LINE OF TIME

Past → Present Moment → **Future**

We are always moving from past to future.

THE POINT OF TIME

Past → **Present Moment** ← Future

The present moment represents all moments.

People living with Alzheimer's tend more and more to experience a point rather than the line of time. Someone might talk about a long-dead relative as if he were just about to arrive for a visit. Or a daughter of sixty is seen as a sister of thirty. It is as if past experience and the future have drawn together with the present as one; much like how our unconscious minds combine several dimensions of time and place when we dream. The present moment represents all moments.

People who meditate regularly—no matter what particular brand of meditation they practice—strive to be in the present moment. In our daily lives our minds are always churning with thoughts, as we think about things other than what we are dealing with at the moment. When we are washing the dishes we think about a conversation we had earlier in the day, or about something we plan to tell someone the next day. The next day, when we are with the person, we think about next month's vacation. When our bodies are in one place and our minds in another, we don't truly experience the present moment. We drive down a street thinking about an appointment we are about to go to, only to realize that we do not remember anything specific about the street we just traveled along. And when we get to the appointment, we worry about how we are going to deal with the results of the meeting, so we aren't really at the meeting—our bodies are there but not our minds. Meditation plays a role in most self-improvement, spiritual, and religious practices. Meditation practice focused on breathing can lead to our being increasingly present to where we actually are, so that our bodies and minds are in the same place at the same time.

Breathing is being; without breath there is no being. The closest experience we can have to actually being in the present moment—that fleeting moment that is gone the moment we experience it—is being totally present to our own breath. When we breathe in and say to ourselves, "Now I am breathing in," and then breathe out following our breath and say to ourselves, "Now I am breathing out," we are present to our own being. This is the closest possible experience to being where we are, or for our minds to be where our bodies are. It is also the closest we can be to being in the mind of a person living with Alzheimer's.

Being in the present moment in meditation sounds strikingly

similar to the way people living with Alzheimer's often experience time—as I've said, this is as a point, not a line. Those who experience time as a line—generally considered "normal"—work hard to forget the regrets they have about the past, and put aside their worries about the future that they cannot control. At the same time they often urge those living with Alzheimer's to replace their experience of time as a "point" by searching for past memories and thinking about the future. The irony of this situation is mind-boggling. The dilemma, and the contradiction, of these inverse "diseases"—Alzheimer's on the one hand and anxiety about the past and future on the other—are brought together through meditation—a practice that we can all engage in to better our understanding of one another.

Mindfulness and *compassion* are two habits and states of mind associated with meditation practice. Mindfulness is the state of being present to others—to nature, animals, ourselves, and to the connection among all of these. With compassion we are not only present to the situation in which others find themselves, we also care about others as we care about ourselves. Compassion encompasses everyone. For people living with Alzheimer's, both states of mind are normal and usual. Awareness of these capacities provides us with peace of mind and with important insights for finding the key to connection with those living with Alzheimer's.

A GUIDED ALZHEIMER'S MEDITATION

This type of meditation begins with sitting quietly on a cushion or chair, with one hand over the other, eyes slightly open and looking down, and breathing naturally from your belly. That's if you are going to meditate alone.

Partners who practice meditating together can develop even greater closeness. The following breathing exercise takes ten to fifteen minutes and, followed once a day, helps relax and center both partners—enabling mindfulness and compassion. Two partners can do this sitting facing each other, knees almost touching, and holding both hands. Or you can sit next to each other, holding the hand closest to the other, or just with folded hands; whatever works best. Partners can both say the words silently to themselves, if both remember them, or one person can say the guiding terms out loud. Writing the key words in large black letters on a single white sheet of paper and placing it between the two partners helps both remember the sequence. Whichever position you choose together, start with both feet on the floor, your back straight, your eyes slightly open and lowered toward the floor, breathing in and out three or four times.

Breathing in and breathing out mindfully provides us the opportunity to remember ourselves without thinking about who we are, where we are, or what we may be worried about. As we breathe in and breathe out, we say silently to ourselves with each in-breath, "Now I am breathing in," and with each out-breath, "Now I am breathing out."

Flower fresh: The popular and almost universally negative images presented of people living with Alzheimer's are hurtful and stand in the way of our healing. Thich Nhat Hanh points out that in paintings the Buddha is often portrayed sitting on a lotus flower. Symbolically, this represents the idea that each of us is light and fresh as a flower no matter where we are; that the negative images we hold of ourselves keep us from achieving our true potential. Every moment that we replace our negative self-image with a picture of ourselves flowering, we awaken to and are renewed in our special qualities—something really important to do when living with Alzheimer's. This set of breathing practices therefore is to say silently to ourselves as we breathe in, "I feel like a flower," and breathing out, "The flower is fresh and alive"—or simply breathe in "Flower" and breathe out "Fresh."

Being here: The suffering we feel living with Alzheimer's, either as the person with the disease or as their partner, comes from regretting the mistakes we feel we have made in the past, and from worrying about what will happen to us in the future. Aware that we are living with Alzheimer's forever we ask, "Why didn't we take that vacation or spend more time with the children?" Or, "What troubles and disappointments will we face in the coming years?" People living with Alzheimer's must therefore be mindful of being in the present where past regrets and future worries can't overwhelm us. Breathing in we feel the present and say silently to ourselves, "Being." Breathing out we say quietly to ourselves, "Here."

Needing help. Partners living with Alzheimer's need help and compassion. This illness is bigger than anyone ought to have to cope with alone. While needing to reach out, at the same time each of us has a natural instinct and skill to help others. Compassion encompasses both taking care of others and seeing that one's own needs are responded to. To express those needs we need to ask for help. In asking for help from others we acknowledge our basic humanity, our helplessness, and our need. In offering others support we feel strong, vital, and useful because we are returning what we have received. This meditation is: Breathing in, we accept that we need help from others in a single word, "needing." Breathing out, we voice the cry for what we need with the single word "help."

Giving love. Living with Alzheimer's is lonely. Partners feel abandoned by the one they love; the person living with the illness feels more and more isolated in thoughts and memories. Love opens both partner and person with the illness, to see and feel new emotions and abilities that Alzheimer's brings. Both people are increasingly able to love and be loved, an ability all of us aspire to and can be mindful of throughout our lives. In Alzheimer's, partners who stay connected to each other do so by reaching inside to say "I love you" and meaning it without reservation and without conditions. Being mindful of the importance of mutual love, we breathe in, saying silently, "Giving," and breathe out, saying silently, "Love."

Growing still. With all the talk of there being no cure for Alzheimer's disease, it is easy to give up. But being able to live a life with quality for the rest of our days is cause for hope. Knowing that the way people talk to each other can help us avoid becoming upset, knowing that the way the environment is organized can help us avoid getting lost, and knowing that the way our days are planned can help us avoid becoming agitated—all are cause for hope. The last meditation reminds us that there are still opportunities for growth and that Alzheimer's is treatable as long as we are determined to better our lives and to keep going. We remember this when we breathe in, saying silently, "Growing," and breathe out, saying silently, "Still."

At the end of each meditation it is helpful to return to remembering ourselves. Breathing in, saying silently, "I know I am breathing in," then breathing out, saying quietly, "I know I am breathing out"—or simply "in" and "out"—accomplishes this.

The following key words serve as a guide to this meditation:

- *In–Out*
- *Flower–Fresh*

- *Being–Here*
- *Needing–Help*
- *Giving–Love*
- *Growing–Still*
- *In–Out*

Practicing mindfulness and compassion is a cornerstone to moving through life's passage that is Alzheimer's, and building the vibrant and loving relationships that yield its gifts.

ACKNOWLEDGMENTS

Many friends, colleagues, and family members played significant roles in making this book a reality. I owe them my thanks. Of course any mistakes are my own.

Jacqueline C. Vischer, who convinced me that I didn't need to write eleven books—just one book with eleven robust chapters.

Sean Caulfield, whose insight into the use of art as Alzheimer's treatment is unparalleled.

Sue Blackler, who demonstrates every day how the approaches in this book actually work.

Sharon Johnson, whose dreams for this book are even greater than mine.

Dan Colucci, who proved that the ideas in this book are practical tools that can sustain themselves in the real world.

Kerry Mills, who embodies the next generation of caring and compassion.

Joan Hyde, who introduced me to the engaging field of Alzheimer's.

Bill Keane, who was practicing the Hearthstone Way before Hearthstone existed.

Cameron Camp, whose ideas mirror mine so much that people think we have worked together for years (we haven't).

Paul Raia, who, in his modesty, teaches everyone what it means to listen and to be present to people living with Alzheimer's.

Robin Orr, whose friendship, counsel, and conversation about compassion have carried me through moments of doubt.

Sally Arteseros, whose editing made sense out of successive initial drafts.

Alice Martell, who, in her toughness, saw the sense and tenderness of the book and made sure it did not get lost.

Jeff Galas, whose insightful editing turned this book into an intriguing story.

Kevin Charras, whose friendship, support, and conversation around the ideas in this book made them clearer to me than they had been.

Cindy Barotte, who plunged into implementing the ideas presented in this book in France, demonstrating that the principles are not culture-bound.

Anne Basting, who lives art and Alzheimer's, and has so much to contribute.

Mary Ellen Geist, who, in caring for her father, let me know how important it is for me to share my ideas.

Marily Cintra, who teaches by living a life in which art and health are merged.

Richard Taylor, whose constant voice for psychosocial treatments and research provided a beacon to aim for.

Ladi Volicer, who brings a significant scientist's view to non-pharmacological treatment.

Joyce Simard, whose open mind and joyous approach to the Alzheimer's journey—especially its end—is inspiring.

Catherine McBride, a role model par excellence, and her husband and constant support, Owen.

Jiska Cohen-Mansfield, who understands profoundly the relationship between environment and the way people living with Alzheimer's react.

John Killick, who lives the principles of this book and makes poetry.

Janet Reno, who showed me that to practice the principles in this book can require profound personal courage.

Cristiane D'Andrea, who saw and believed and built.

Cindy Hecht, who understands the power of ideas and spreading the word.

ARTZ artists-in-residence Tanya Azarani, who led the way by being the first; Cat Cuthillo, whose dedication to photographing events was inspiring; Dalmoni Lydijusse, who taught us that even a gentle response is a meaningful response; and Lauren Volkmer, whose embrace of art for Alzheimer's was life-changing.

Gary Glazner, whose enthusiasm and insight bring joy to those he touches with poetry.

All the institutions and organizations that embraced ARTZ and helped promote this important concept: the Louvre (Mathieu Decraine); the Museum of Modern Art, New York; the National Gallery of Australia, Canberra; Tribeca Film Institute; Cirque Phénix; the Bowery Poetry Club; Big Apple Circus (Paul Binder, Mike Christianson, Andrea Koppel); and the National Arts Club.

Dianne Davis, who is actively promoting international recognition of the ARTZ museum program.

Julie Winter, who was willing at the drop of a hat to meditate with people living with Alzheimer's.

Denis Phelouzat, who understands the poetry of architecture that works for people.

Igor Tojcic, who has steadfastly put himself on the line to

bring the ideas in this book into practice in the NHS in Barnet and London.

Mark Nemschoff, who selflessly supported the first ARTZ exhibition.

Henry McCance, who saw the value of both genetics research and the ARTZ Museum Partnership in Massachusetts.

Wayne Ruga, who showed me that without a book the word would remain inert.

Frank Ertola, Sheila Barnes, Irene and Myron Benson, Wolf Goldstein, and Reuben Rosen, whose enthusiasm and caring showed us the way.

Sister Dang Nghiem, who resolved with grace the last phrase of the meditation.

Albert Low, who introduced me to the power of meditation.

Meredith Patterson, whose support of the Hearthstone Way goes beyond geriatric care management.

Maureen Matthews, who blends creativity, caring, and playwriting.

Olivier Drunat and Joel Belmin, leading the way of non-pharmacological treatment in France.

Michèle Fremontier and the Médéric Foundation, fighting the good fight in France.

Jean Radvanyi and Annie Radzinski, whose continued support and interest in my work helped me develop the precision of my ideas.

Ruvani Da Silva, who heard a radio interview in Sydney and called.

Cornelia Beck, whose straightforward research approach puts nonpharmacological treatment into the everyday—an important step.

Michelle Bourgeois, whose enthusiasm for all we do is infectious.

Bonnie LaMothe, who sees the future and is making it happen.

Cheryl and Derek Markham, who have planted and are watering the seeds of the *I'm Still Here* approach in Australia.

Jonathan Leiserach, who recommended I read Stephen King's *On Writing*.

Paul Robertson, who taught me that music is too precise for words.

Sezgin Kaya, whose intellectual curiousity, advice, and unwavering support have helped me refine my thinking immeasurably.

John Eberhard, whose leadership of the Academy of Neuroscience for Architecture (ANFA) opened significant doors and whose wise counsel remains always welcome.

Barry Reisberg, whose early articles identified the power of nonpharmacological approaches to reduce behavioral symptoms of Alzheimer's.

REFERENCES

Books and Articles

Alexander, Christopher. *The Timeless Way of Building.* New York: Oxford University Press, 1979.

Arnheim, Rudolf. *Art and Visual Perception: A Psychology of the Creative Eye.* Berkeley: University of California Press, 1954.

Basting, Anne. *Timeslips: Creative Storytelling with People with Dementia.* Milwaukee: UWM-Milwaukee Center on Aging and Community, 2004.

Bayley, John. *Elegy for Iris.* New York: Picador, USA, 1999.

Calkins, Magaret. *Design for Dementia: Planning Environments for the Elderly and the Confused.* Owings Mills, MD: National Health Publishing, 1988.

Camp, Cameron J. "Montessori-Based Dementia Programming™ in Long-Term Care: A Case Study of Disseminating an Intervention for Persons with Dementia." In R. C. Intrieri and L. Hyer, eds., *Clinical Applied Gerontological Interventions in Long-term Care,* pp. 295–314. New York: Springer, 2006.

Camp, Cameron J. "Spaced Retrieval: A Case Study in Dissemination of a Cognitive Intervention for Persons with Dementia." In D. Koltai Attix and Kathleen A. Welsch-Bohmner, eds., *Geriatric Neuropsychological Assessment and Intervention.* pp. 275–292. New York: Guilford, 2006.

Changeux, Jean-Pierre. *Neuronal Man: The Biology of Man.* Trans. Laurence Garey. Princeton, NJ: Princeton University Press, 1985.

Cohen, Uriel, and Gerald Weisman. *Holding On to Home: Designing Environments for People with Dementia.* Baltimore: The Johns Hopkins University Press, 1991.

Cohen-Mansfield, Jiska, and Perla Werner. "Environmental Influences on Agitation: An Integrative Summary of an Observational Study." *The American Journal of Alzheimer's Care & Related Disorders and Research,* vol. 10, no. 1 (1995), pp. 32–39.

Damasio, Antonio R. *Descartes' Error: Emotion, Reason, and the Human Brain.* New York: G. P. Putnam's Sons, 1994.

Doherty, Brian. "A Visit to Wyeth Country." In Wanda M. Corn, *The Art of Andrew Wyeth,* pp. 14–43. Boston: Little, Brown, 1973.

Ekman, Paul. *Emotions Revealed: Recognizing Faces and Feelings to Improve Communication and Emotional Life.* New York: Times Books, 2003.

Emerson Lombardo, N. B., L. Volicer, A. Martin, B. Wu and X. W. Zhang. "Memory Preservation Diet to Reduce Risk and Slow Progression of Alzheimer's Disease." In B. Vellas, M. Grundman, H. Feldman, L. J. Fitten, and B. Winblad, eds., *Research and Practice in Alzheimer's Disease and Cognitive Decline,* vol. 9: pp. 138–159.

Gazzaniga, Michael S. *The Mind's Past.* Berkeley: University of California Press, 1998.

Gladwell, Malcolm. *The Tipping Point: How Little Things Can Make a Big Difference*. Boston: Little, Brown, 2000.

Glazner, Gary. *Sparking Memories: The Alzheimer's Poetry Project Anthology*. Santa Fe, NM: Poem Factory, 2005.

Kandel, Eric R. *In Search of Memory: The Emergence of a New Science of Mind*. New York: W. W. Norton, 2006.

Killick, John, and Carl Cordonner, eds. *Openings: Dementia Poems and Photographs,* London: Hawker, 2000.

Kitwood, Tom. *Dementia Reconsidered: The Person Comes First*. London: Open University Press, 1997.

Lawton, M. Powell. "Environmental Approaches to Research and Treatment of Alzheimer's Disease." In E. Light and B. D. Lebowitz, eds. *Treatment and Family Stress: Direction for Research*. Bethesda, MD: National Institute of Mental Health, U.S. Department of Health and Human Services, 1990.

Leviten, Daniel J. *This Is Your Brain on Music: The Science of a Human Obsession*. New York: Plume, 2007.

Lorenz, Konrad, with Michael Martys and Angelika Tipler. *Here Am I— Where Are You: The Behavior of the Greylag Goose*. Trans. Robert D. Martin, New York: Harcourt Brace Jovanovich, 1991.

Lynch, Kevin. *The Image of the City*. Cambridge, MA: The MIT Press, 1960.

Mace, Nancy, and Peter Rabins. *The 36-Hour Day*. Baltimore: The Johns Hopkins University Press, 1981.

Mahoney, E. K., Ladislav Volicer, and Ann C. Hurley. *Management of Challenging Behaviors in Dementia*. Baltimore: Health Professions, 2000.

McBride, Cathleen. "Setting a New Stage." Alzheimer's Association Massachusetts Chapter, newsletter, vol. 21, no. 3 (2003), p. 10.

Merton, Robert K. *Social Theory and Social Structure*. New York: Free Press, 1957.

Moberg, Kersten Uvnas. *The Oxytocin Factor: Tapping the Hormone of Calm, Love, and Healing*. Cambridge, MA: Da Capo, 2003.

Montessori, Maria. *The Secret of Childhood*. New York: Ballantine, 1966.

Nhat Hanh, Thich. *Nothing to Do, Nowhere to Go.* Berkeley, CA: Parallax, 2007.

Norman, Donald A. *The Design of Everyday Things.* New York: Doubleday/Currency, 1990.

Orr, Robin. "Compassion and the Healthcare Industry." Keynote speech, Center for Health Design Conference, Chicago, 2007.

Raia, Paul. "Sleuthing Troublesome Behaviors à la Sherlock Holmes." Alzheimer's Association, Massachusetts Chapter, newsletter, vol. 23, no. 2 (2005), pp. 1–7.

Ramachandran, V. S., and Sandra Blakeslee. *Phantoms in the Brain: Probing the Mysteries of the Human Mind.* New York: William Morrow, 1998.

Reisberg, Barry, et al. "Evidence and Mechanisms of Retrogenesis in Alzheimer's and Other Dementias: Management and Treatment Import." *American Journal of Alzheimer's Disease,* vol. 17 (2002), pp. 202–212.

Rowe, John W., and Robert L. Kahn. *Successful Aging.* New York: Dell, 1998.

Salzberg, Sharon, and Jon Kabat-Zinn. "Mindfulness as Medicine." In Daniel Goleman, ed., *Healing Emotions: Conversations with the Dalai Lama on Mindfulness, Emotions, and Health,* pp. 107–144. Boston and London: Shambala, 2003.

Schacter, Daniel L. *Searching for Memory: The Brain, the Mind, and the Past.* New York: Basic Books, 1996.

Taylor, Richard. *Alzheimer's from the Inside Out.* Baltimore: Health Professions, 2007.

Teresa, Mother. *Meditations from a Simple Path.* New York: Ballantine, 1996.

Teri, Linda, Laura E. Gibbons, Susan M. McCurry, Rebecca G. Logsdon, David M. Buchner, William E. Barlow, Walter A. Kukull, Andrea Z. LaCroix, Wayne McCormick, and Eric B. Larson. "Exercise Plus Behavioral Management in Patients with Alzheimer's Disease: A Randomized Controlled Trial." *Journal of the American Medical Association,* vol. 290, no. 15 (2003), pp. 2015–2022.

Volicer, Ladislav. "Treatment of Behavioral Disorders." In J. Pathy, A. J. Sinclair, and J. E. Morley, eds., *Principles and Practice of Geriatric Medicine,* pp. 1135–1148. Chichester, England: John Wiley & Sons, 2006.

Volicer, Ladislav, and Lisa Bloom-Charette, *Enhancing the Quality of Life in Advanced Dementia.* New York: Taylor & Francis, 1999.

Volicer, Ladislav, and Ann C. Hurley. "Management of Behavioral Symptoms in Progressive Degenerative Dementias." *Journal of Gerontology: Medical Sciences,* vol. 58A (2003), pp. 837–845.

Whitehouse, Peter J., with Daniel George. *The Myth of Alzheimer's: What You Aren't Being Told About Today's Most Dreaded Diagnosis.* New York: St. Martin's Press, 2008.

Zeisel, John. "Creating a Therapeutic Garden That Works for People Living with Alzheimer's." In Susan Rodiek and Benyamin Schwartz, eds., *Outdoor Environments for People with Dementia.* Binghamton, NY: Hayworth, 2007.

Zeisel, John. "Healing Gardens for People Living with Alzheimer's: Challenges to Creating an Evidence Base for Treatment Outcomes." In Catherine Ward Thompson, ed., *Open Space: People Space.* London: Taylor & Francis, 2007.

Zeisel, John. *Inquiry by Design: Environment/Behavior/Neuroscience in Architecture, Interiors, Landscape and Planning.* Rev. ed. New York: W. W. Norton, 2006.

Zeisel, John. "Life-Quality Alzheimer Care in Assisted Living." In Benjamin Schwartz and Ruth Brent, eds., *Aging, Autonomy, and Architecture: Advances in Assisted Living.* Baltimore: The Johns Hopkins University Press, 1999.

Zeisel, John. "Universal Design to Support the Brain and Its Development." In Wolfgang F. E. Preiser and Elaine Ostroff, eds., *Universal Design Handbook.* New York: McGraw-Hill, 2001.

Zeisel, John, Joan Hyde, and Susan Levkoff. "Best Practices: An Environment-Behavior (E-B) Model for Alzheimer Special Care Units." *American Journal of Alzheimer's Care & Research,* vol. 9, no. 2 (1994), pp. 4–21.

Zeisel, John, and Paul Raia. "Nonpharmacological Treatment for Alzheimer's Disease: A Mind-Brain Approach." *American Journal of Alzheimer's Disease and Other Dementias,* vol. 15, no. 6 (2000), pp. 331–340.

Zeisel, John, Nina M. Silverstein, Joan Hyde, M. Powell Lawton, and William Holmes. "Environmental Correlates to Behavioral Outcomes in Alzheimer's Special Care Units." *The Gerontologist,* vol. 43, no. 5 (October 2003), pp. 687–711.

Zeisel, John, and Martha Tyson. "Alzheimer's Treatment Gardens." In Clare Cooper Marcus and Marni Barnes, eds., *Healing Gardens: Therapeutic Benefits and Design Recommendations.* New York: John Wiley & Sons, 1999.

Websites

The Alzheimer's Association	www.alz.org
Artists for Alzheimer's (ARTZ)	www.artistsforalzheimers.org
Big Apple Circus	www.bigapplecircus.org
Bowery Poetry Club	www.bowerypoetry.com
Hearthstone Alzheimer Care	www.thehearth.org
John Michael Kohler Art Center	www.jmkac.org
Tribeca Film Institute	www.tribecafilminstitute.org

ARTZ: Artists for Alzheimer's is a trademark of the Artists for Alzheimer's program of the Hearthstone Alzheimer's Foundation.

INDEX